The Purple Envelope

The Purple Envelope

ANOTHER SIDE OF CANCER

Vivien Jones

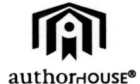

AuthorHouse™
1663 Liberty Drive
Bloomington, IN 47403
www.authorhouse.com
Phone: 1-800-839-8640

© 2011 by Vivien Jones. All rights reserved.

No part of this book may be reproduced, stored in a retrieval system, or transmitted by any means without the written permission of the author.

First published by AuthorHouse   07/26/2011

ISBN: 978-1-4567-8436-2 (sc)
ISBN: 978-1-4567-8437-9 (ebk)

Printed in the United States of America

Any people depicted in stock imagery provided by Thinkstock are models, and such images are being used for illustrative purposes only.
Certain stock imagery © Thinkstock.

This book is printed on acid-free paper.

Because of the dynamic nature of the Internet, any web addresses or links contained in this book may have changed since publication and may no longer be valid. The views expressed in this work are solely those of the author and do not necessarily reflect the views of the publisher, and the publisher hereby disclaims any responsibility for them.

To Welties

This is a story about a family with some main characters – quite ordinary in a way. As in anyone's story this one has some extraordinary moments and the writer is telling them all. If it ever seems to the reader as a bit much, he can know that being ordinary they too found many of the situations and circumstances a bit much, even as they were happening. But they are included here regardless. In the sense that everyone's life is a story, this story is one year of one man's life and the lives of people around him.

Or is it a story of love and how it plays its tune in this young man's life. Is it true? Oh yes, and as such has unbelievable moments. The writer welcomes you, the reader, to her world. Come as a friend or a neighbour. You'll first meet her in England away from cities where its beauty can be called gentle but where life happens in ways that you will recognize wherever you may be. Because it's about people interacting with others, it's a story about that which makes the world go round.

Life's Flight

Fly with me and take the sky
It is now that my life is mine.
I've got this short time on earth
And my longing has brought me here.
All I lacked and all I gained
And yet it's the way that I chose.
My trust was far beyond words
That has shown me a little bit
Of the heaven I've never found.
I want to feel that I'm alive
All my living days
I want to feel that I'm alive,
Knowing it was good enough.

Anon

1

I step out, glad to walk away from long hours at work.

Today I take the direction of the Post Office, the only shop in the hamlet, in remote English countryside. Fran will be behind the counter with friendly chitchat and maybe a batch of scones; once a barmaid, warm, round with marshmallow softness and that ageless gleam in her eye. We share the same birthday. The twenty-four years between us are meaningless in the understanding we share.

Good feelings accompany each step and I take a short cut through the Dower House grounds. Here daffodils grow like rows of trumpets agreeable with the upbeat of my pace and with them, scattered beneath the trees, are soft white feathers which come from who knows where.

There's no chance today to reach the nearby town with its selection of greeting cards.

Not today the two-mile walk across the fields of recently germinating crops where I enjoy the sun dappled farm footpath. Always the breeze adds movement and energy to the walk. Birdcalls must be at their sweetest here in this natural corner of Kent – sometimes dubbed the garden of England. Instead, through the Dower House grounds where the Lord's widow resides as the young Lord and his family take their place in the Manor House.

With limited time today I take this short cut to the single local shop – the old Post Office. I reach for the antique door handle and chimes without melody jingle as I step into the small shop. Pictures of local aristocracy adorn the walls – the gamekeeper at his lodge – the Lord and Lady of the manor in whose park-like grounds I'm free to meander for these hours that I'm free from work.

But today, Michael is on my mind. Michael. I soundlessly shape his name and my tongue lingers at the roof of my mouth. His arrival, so long after our pigeon pair, was a gift and now he's about to leave his teen years behind. Typically I think of his childhood, extravagantly aware that he's ready for adulthood. Back in Johannesburg my last child, born much later than the others, will get my card in April, just before my return.

The sound of Fran's shuffle from her adjoining cottage comes to me with the smell of fresh baking; then her cheery call to be patient as at 81 she makes her entrance through the heavy curtain dividing duty from domesticity. Her stick thumps a dead beat on floorboards belying the vitality she brings into the room.

I turn, expecting and wanting to receive warmth from her smiling eyes. We are pals agreeing not to gossip and we laugh easily just because it's a good life we live.

I am already scanning the cards on display and her glance goes to the birthday card in my hand . . . which to choose? My thoughts toy with the choice tuning out her chatter about expected deliveries of cards soon, and soon-to-be-ready fresh baked scones. That's her special welcome for each of her maybe dozen customers a day.

The Purple Envelope

My thoughts are six thousand miles away. They are with Michael in Helderkruin in South Africa.

Which one . . . which card . . .

The card with the fishing rod, sailing boat, long low red car would do. Would he one day have these things I wonder, and while pondering I remember his first car – a reliable old model which had left enough in his budget for flying lessons.

I smile. With his twentieth birthday celebration he'll celebrate getting his license to fly a microlight. My stare shifts to the second card I hold in my hands . . . a card with a light aircraft. The caption reads "A Man in a Million".

Well, that says it!

I am his mother and a man in a million is what he is; but I hesitate seeing its envelope, remembering how often mail is lost in transit to South Africa. A purple envelope invites curiosity. A purple envelope will give away the personal nature of its contents.

The sports car, boat and fishing-rod card is returned to the rack and, still disturbed by the risk, I hold the purple envelope and stroke to feel the texture of recycled paper. I run my finger along its folded edge resting at one blunt corner.

Many hands will hold it before it gets to its destination. Is it too much of a risk? Its loss, its fate if handled by thieving shifty fingers, has no material importance but great personal meaning.

I am aware of silence. Fran has stopped talking, sensing my preoccupation. I run my finger down the price list, hand her the coins. The card is chosen and my own words will add to the printed verse while Fran retreats beyond the curtain to bring the promised scones and Earl Grey tea.

I write:

> *I wish you a life in which you fly*
> *In which you soar in all your endeavours.*
> *Happy Birthday always Mom. X X*

I read it and wonder if I've spelt endeavour right. Wish I was there with him for that day.

I add underneath superfluously,

> *Will see you soon after your birthday*

It is done. The address in place; stamp affixed, I slip it into the slit of one of the oldest post boxes in existence. Purple out of sight now, I look at the old-fashioned royal red post box. Have to touch it – run my finger over the ornamentation as many have before me.

Back inside, I take the tray from Fran.

No more doubts about the card. Trust. Butter melts into feather light scone. Homemade strawberry jam tops it and hot tea enhances an already perfect day.

The only interruption happens at mid-day. The Postman arrives and empties the mail box. He looks young – too young, but cheerfully whistles through his day. Fran takes a chocolate down from a shelf for him and he grins walking out casually, leaving us to chatter with the jangle of door chimes in the air.

* * *

In South Africa, Michael at his desk is intent on creating solutions. He was out celebrating his friends 21st last night – a long time friend from early childhood, and he stayed partying until the early hours. It left few hours for sleep but, with what even he recognizes as probably too much optimism, he thinks he'll catch up.

At work, the company is not sure that they'll meet their deadline and Michael will stay late and find some fast food nearby to take care of a meal. That way he can call by the flying club and see how the service maintenance is going. Once the used microlight that he wants to buy has got its air-worthy certificate, he'll be sure of a hanger space lease.

His mates will have a practice run tonight, but this time he'll forego the extra preparation for the weekend's long distance run. He'll call instead at the gym to coincide with Clare being there. He can see her on Friday as well and still have the assignment finished and sent out in good time on Monday morning. The B Com correspondence course is time-taking but he wants to keep it up.

Ah, he could hear the drinks trolley on the corridor – the rumble comes ahead of Joey's arrival, signalling the routine morning break. His dry humour and cavalier attitude amuse Michael and he sends a comic remark his way. At this company free soda is supplied and that's a cool thing about working here. Michael buys two packets of chips and tosses the empty cola can into a container under his desk. He has a reason for keeping them but I'm not sure what it is.

For the first time in hours he leans back in his chair and stretches out feeling he is pretty much on top of his part of the project, but you could never tell until it went live. Heads turn in his direction as the cell phone on his desk starts ringing. It plays Wallace and Grommet's theme tune rather too loudly. He enjoys it; enjoys his life. On the line is someone who is guiding him into some investment – small stuff, but a start.

His thoughts drift to his mother who is away working in England. He will talk to her at the weekend about a house she's looking for. He thinks about taking her for a flight when she's at home again.

The call over, his attention is immediately focused back on the task at hand.

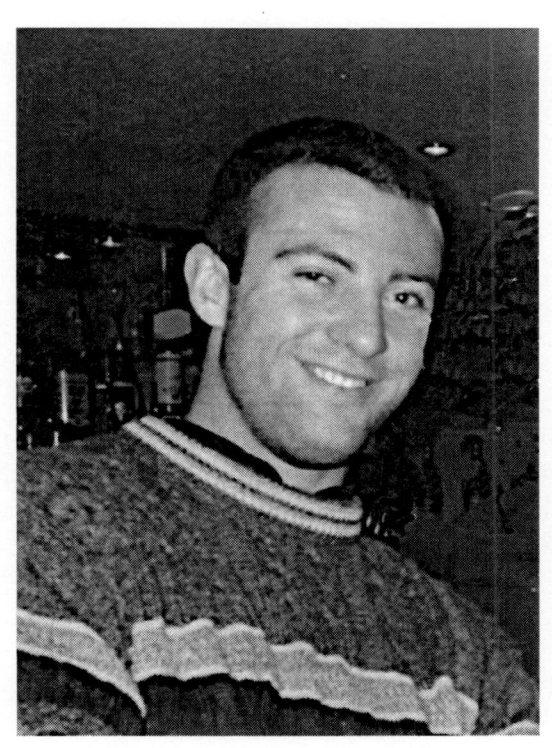

2

> Love is something eternal,
> the aspect may change
> but not the essence.
> Vincent van Gogh

It's August now and I've returned to England from South Africa. Between work assignments with different aged people, I search out a cottage for myself. I am regularly assigned as a companion to, and have grown fond of, Mrs Platt the doctor's widow; of gracious Freda Neete; and of the admiral that I could only call admirable.

The worn cottage that would be my home during the times I was in England was essentially at the lower end of the market. The small place would suit my needs and I was game for the renovating.

The one I settled for that summer in 2001 was not inspiring then. Some renovation and modernization had already been done but it still needed work to bring it up to a standard that would make it cute, or quaint and cottagey. But it was affordable and the only structural repair was minimal – just something in the loft around the chimney needed attention – or did it need a new chimney!

The approach to this Somerset cottage was an open courtyard laid with scattered shingle for parking. The area was rather smaller than necessary to properly accommodate the few cars owned by the inhabitants of the eight terrace houses. The garden was separate from the house. It was obviously from days gone by when a garden was not so much a play-area or aesthetic backdrop for a house, as a patch for growing vegetables. This patch had the washing line, a small shed for garden tools, and a garden chair.

The decision to purchase had been difficult because of my lifestyle – I was not always in the country. The next of my frequent trips to South Africa was due and there was limited time to attend to everything before then. I had a long overdue trip to Canada to fit in which would further delay my return. It was unavoidable that I would be away for longer than usual this time. I talked it over with my family and had their full support.

And so, it's mid August and I'm working in Bushton at the Admiral's extensive seaside house. We breakfast together at the knotty pine kitchen table and I'm glad I got the boiled egg right, cooking it to his instructions. He dips a finger of well-buttered bread first into salt and then soft yolk and skilfully avoids an overflow. Satisfied, he looks up with an approving nod.

"I'll check the newspaper before taking a swim."

At eighty six his eyes can read only headlines and his thick black marker ticks articles of interest. He is impatient to know the remainder so I read it out before we prepare for pool exercises. Then in the pool we methodically run through a routine. With a sweep of his hand he indicates that I may swim on – he'll wait in the nursery. His strong robed form disappears. I enjoy the water, swimming at my own pace. With the aged, things happen at a slow pace.

Towelling myself before joining him in the nursery, Michael comes to mind, and my other son Anthony. All is well in South Africa. Yes, all is well and I try to shrug off some vague doubt as being a mother's excessive concern. I tell myself not to be silly.

But I am not silly. I know they are fine but something is clouding my sense of peace. The cross continents phone chats always reassure me so this growing cloud is to be dismissed. I am excited about my life.

Soon I will own a cottage in an English country village. My phone rings and I hear the cool voice of the estate agent's representative confirm that papers for the deal will be faxed to the local city internet café today.

Faxing is safe, I muse. Snail mail can disappoint . . . e-mails are instant and the connection often confirmed with immediacy like being in conversation. But snail mail has a personal touch, like greetings cards that have been passed from hand to hand until finally reaching the recipient's hand. Even before opening, its arrival says "I thought of you" and that is what I had hoped the purple envelope would say.

It is four months since Michael's twentieth birthday, and still from time to time I ask him if the card in the purple envelope has arrived. I'm ever hopeful, but I have to accept the reality. My greeting was lost – or intercepted – in transit. We wonder if it was a statistical loss, or may it have been thieving by someone hoping to find an inserted gift. How pointless! It's just not enough for him to know that I

The Purple Envelope

wrote. His birthday came and went with an empty space between us.

I was at home with him for three weeks before returning to work in England. As I left, two friends moved in with Michael for the duration of my absence. Two rugby playing, bright, fun loving, healthy friends who would get their first experience of living away from home. All worked in the IT industry; they were school friends. They were eager for the independence and sometimes I thought I'd like to be a fly on the wall.

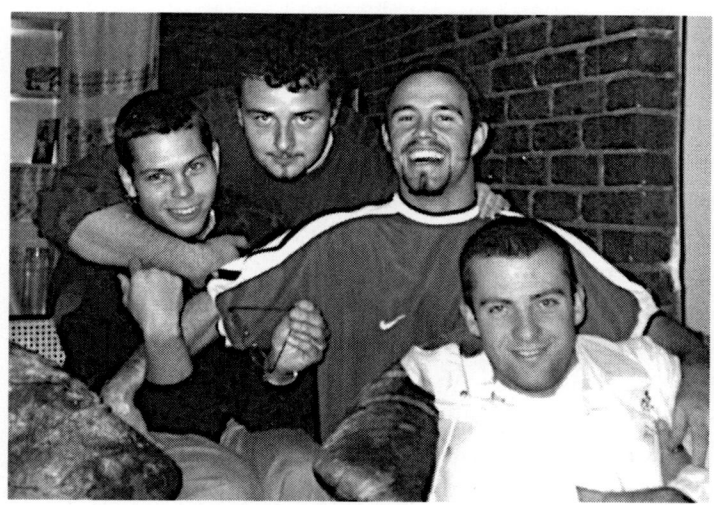

Dion, Daniel, Doug, Michael

His birthday followed a break-up with his girlfriend Clare. A young man growing young love faces love in the future more fragilely than we who have scar tissue where our hearts were wounded.

Why this melancholy! Kisses are blown into cyberspace on e-mail and somehow they are received across the world. How is that!

The Rear Admiral wants a drive out today. It should be fun although my favourites with him are the walks in the woods or along the beach that skirts his grounds. I engage the gear of his ridiculously old vehicle and pull into the drive. The tarmac runs under servants bedrooms that span between the main house and the garages. It amuses him to make it a mystery tour.

"Turn left . . . right next . . . onto the farm track".

So we go. I am lost; he's in charge. The countryside is fresh after recent summer showers and we prolong being there.

"May we detour for a stop at the cyber cafe to pick up a fax?"

I'm confident he won't mind and can't wait to proceed with this deal – to own the quaint two-bedroom cottage in Somerset.

"No," he says.

"*What!*" I think.

"Let's get back."

He wanted to get back. Surprising, but there it was. We sailed past the cyber café route and drove straight home – home to his daughters who were visiting for tea. Their visit gave me the opportunity to slip out and I asked Sally if she would give me thirty minutes while they chatted. She was happy to oblige.

My car sped to town. It was ten minutes to get there, five minutes for my business and ten minutes back . . . back to give medication in good time.

The fax had arrived but the sweet lady helping me couldn't see where it was. She searched in drawers and

The Purple Envelope

through a file. She scratched in the waste bin and checked drawers again. Shaking her head she said repeatedly how sorry she was and looked around for her assistant (who had slipped out for a chocolate) for ideas of where else to look.

I saw a parking space on the road-side and excused myself. I ran across to where I had hastily parked in the railway car park and brought my car up to the shop front where the free space was mercifully still empty.

I thought the problem would have sorted itself out by then, but no such good fortune.

I might as well see if there was mail for me while I waited. I wandered over to a computer and logged on. A surprising e mail from Emily came up. It went like this:

> The middle verse in the Bible is Psalm 118 v 8
> 594 verses lead up to it and 594 verses follow it
> 594 and 594 add up to 1188.

How like my daughter to keep in touch in this way.

She went on, "Mum that verse at the heart of the Bible says, rather than having confidence in men, put your trust in God".

Hmm that's nice . . . with the numbers like that!

At that moment, the sweet lady hurried over to me. She had a crumpled fax paper in her hands. Quite flushed, she explained she'd found it in the waste bin. She was flattening it against her skirt as she spoke.

As I drove home, I thought of the day's happenings. Timing made the events of the afternoon what they were. It was Sally's arrival for tea which allowed me, during working hours, to leave for the city. As luck would have it, parking was impossible and being required to be back within half an hour was the constraint that persuaded me to make the unlawful turn into the station car park. A heavy fine was the penalty, but I risked it. A jog across to the café and the errand would be completed quickly, I had thought until the fax bringing details of the cottage could not be found. Thankfully, a space for my car became vacant outside the shop.

Yes timing made the events of the afternoon what they were. The delay caused by the missing fax had allowed me to see Emily's email, I mused as I drove along the private road to the admiral's coastal home, my mind still running over the difficulties that had made that simple errand stressful.

A letter is on the mat as I step inside the hallway. I stoop to pick it up and notice again the dramatic swirls of his sister's handwriting that as always cover most of the ochre envelope and I notice, for the first time, that the postal code ends with 1188.

"I do trust," I think, but I am soon to learn to trust much more.

We spend the evening with Mozart and Beethoven and while listening to exquisite music, I quell eagerness to examine the details of the cottage until my charge is settled in bed. You never know if later on in the small hours, his over-use of barbiturates, started in World War 2's bombing raids, will provoke a nightmare and so interrupt the night hours for us both.

Back in my room, for once I don't linger at the window where I can view the seascape. The yacht club's crafts can be seen amid hardly rippling water as they're under just enough moonlight.

I peruse the fax. The repair to the chimney is small. 170 year old places like it are still around. My attention is caught by the last number of the village's postal code. There it is – this time 188.

Trust God.

I retire to bed content with my life and the prospect of this home.

* * *

It's Sunday evening and I get through to Michael with a call to his mobile phone. The mobile number is listed in my travel diary alongside his office number and my glance takes it in. It is something that hasn't meant anything before, but now there's a startling coincidence in seeing the office number which ends 0188.

" . . . really, there's nothing for you to worry about Mom, enjoy yourself."

His voice reaches my consciousness from six thousand miles away, in spite of the distraction of seeing that number.

"Yes, work is going well but we're very busy, so I am working extra hours," he told me.

His friends were happy in the flat.

"The cooking is great and we're OK with the laundry too," he said.

"So everything's alright," I stated.

"Yes, nothing to worry about," he sounded as he always did.

These children of mine were too concerned that I should have an untroubled life and enjoy this time away with people I grew up with while revisiting haunts of my childhood.

Nothing in his voice gave a clue to either settle or confirm my unease. After all, it was instinct that told me to be concerned.

"If I was there, would I think everything's alright, that there's nothing to worry about?" My voice was passive, lightly phrased to cut through any sense that he had to prove himself. Sure he was able to look after himself. But this wasn't about that. I had a mother's inkling of something not being right.

The silence in the phone's earpiece gave a clear answer that I'd touched a chord.

The call ended cheerfully and I returned to my tasks, and he to his life with two flat mates.

He had been a bit nauseous and had put it down to a simple stomach bug. It started with vomiting soon after eating. He would see the doctor and have it checked out.

In his office on Monday morning, Michael leaned back in his office chair stretching out with hands behind his head. He ran his hand across his lower chest and stopped suddenly . . . what was that? Hard like rubber – below his rib cage – like a tyre? Muscle? He'd like to think so but . . . he phoned the doctor and made an appointment for later that day.

3

My bags are packed and I'm ready to leave the Admiral in someone else's care the following day. We, his three companions, rotate like this every two weeks.

For one more evening I sit with him tuned to listen to his favourite classical music on high tech equipment. I'm on duty. My presence is all he needs and my mind wanders. The cloud of concern for my family in South Africa is ever present. What is it that nags at my peace?

Before I start the next assignment I have a day's leave. I load my car and lock my temporary home – a beach bothy in the admiral's grounds – before driving forty miles for the new job. There will be time to look round 'A Delightful Muddle'. I like some of the shop's used and antique stuff which may have more English charm than purpose, but my eye is practised at finding gems to store away for use in the cottage. The search was long for a chest of drawers but with time to browse, a small collection of affordable things has grown. I smile remembering how my children sometimes regard my treasures.

"Oh no! Mum's been to the firewood shop again," they groan . . . or are they laughing!

It was well through August and the warm weather complimented my easy sandals-and-t-shirt mood. With time to spare, I went into a book shop and browsed, appreciating the quietness and their good coffee. I looked through the books reduced in price and noticed Chicken Soup for the Soul. I picked it up and turned it over and did that again . . . and then again. It caught my interest so much . . . it would be good to look through but I had enough to read. I finally walked away, out of the shop without it and went on to Southampton where Mrs Platt, a doctors widow, was expecting me.

That's where I was when the call came in.

Our family doctor of many years in Johannesburg, whom Michael saw that day, sent him for x-rays and he first told his brother this news, and he passed it on to Emily in Kent. Seeing my daughter's name announce her incoming call on my cell phone's screen, brightened any day. Far from home a call from any family member was a welcome interlude. This time I heard her say,

"Mum, Michael has a lesion on his stomach."

"A lesion? What is that?"

Michael has a lesion on his stomach. In my mind, I replay what I heard.

Something's attached to Michael's stomach and while it doesn't mean a lot to me, I see concern beneath the demeanour of Mrs Platt's cultured friendliness.

The following day, Wednesday 29th August, the specialist told Michael that he had a cancerous growth in his connective tissue, and this news reached me in the same way.

"Hello Mum," there is natural kindness in Emily's voice.

She used few words. The one that held me was cancer. That's what it was to me, a word – like monsoon. It had bad connotations, but was out of my field of reference. I would have to go . . . be with him until he was over it . . . while he was treated.

The specialist took tissue from his neck gland for laboratory testing to determine the type of growth it was. The biopsy confirmed that it was malignant. They gave it a name but they weren't sure without further tests. Words I was to hear before it was finally identified were: Sarcoma; germ cell cancer; young man's cancer; yolk sac tumour; embryonic cancer – in his connective tissue. There were numerous secondary cannon balls in his lungs. It had metastasised. I wonder what effect that news has on other mothers who hear it for the first time. I couldn't relate. It was an uninvited visitor in my world and had the wrong address. Not us, not Michael. It didn't fit. No!!! No . . .

Cancer.

"It's cancer, Mrs Platt."

"Oh dear!"

How still the quietness was between us.

"Pray. That's all you can do." The way she said it was a prayer.

I sensed deep emotion in her frail countenance and prayerfulness in her tone. I felt gratitude even if I didn't say so. I prepared to go to him. I'd be there while he was treated and cured.

Tanya phoned. She wept. She is a much loved daughter-in-law and she wept saying how sorry she was. She had found out about vitamin B17 and was waiting for a delivery from the States. It wasn't available there in South

Africa. I had some nutritional training and hadn't heard of it. I was later to know a great deal about it.

I drove back to the admiral's bothy which was my home base, but only after Mrs Platt's replacement companion arrived. She came into Southampton railway station. Even without a description, I could pick her out from the small crowd of disembarking travellers. She looked depressed. She looked as if life was more than enough for her to cope with. She was overweight and she looked irritated by the burden of her heavy suitcase.

So confident was I that it was her, that I walked over to meet her. Close up, I saw even better just how beautiful she was under long heavy shapeless hair. How sad that her beauty was hidden under a dull façade.

I took her suitcase.

"It's health food," she said. "I don't eat from the lady's table."

Packet soup with few calories; nutritionally balanced meal replacing powder; low-sugar, or no sugar-content bars of sweets, made up the bulk of her possessions. I thought of the lamb roast I had prepared earlier for her lunch but listened attentively to her story as we rode back. It was a chance that I took, but said some bold things to encourage her to take a peep through a different porthole at life. Whether surprised or not, she heeded it all.

I introduced her to Mrs Platt and left.

On the way to the bothy in Bushton, the phone rang. I pulled in to hear the cool voice of the building society representative confirming that papers were being compiled – formal details for the deal.

I somehow found words to tell her that I couldn't continue with the deal. I was implicitly sorry but it was all too much to take on. She offered me a reduced price – I needed time to think and she said she would fax certain details for me to consider. I was glad of the delay – get back to the bothy and take advantage of the time. My immediate future was uncertain.

I sped along the serious arterial road – marked red on the map but actually only a country road – to my beach-side temporary home.

My thoughts went back to the cottage. I would let that one go and look for a cottage once again when I returned. Delaying that dream was regrettable. The phone call to the estate agent was easy; just a few minutes to change the course that my life would take. The cottage purchase was cancelled. It was done.

At the bothy, with boxes, bubble wrap, and moth balls, I soon have my few things tidily out of the way. For the three or four month absence that I anticipate, this would be enough I determine. But why is there a sense that I am not doing enough. Basics for my cottage are there, the treasures that were fun to find by rummaging in shops like A Delightful Muddle. Other people's remnant items of porcelain became my treasures. The china and glass is stored away in the bothy for the permanent home I will have one day.

Before I leave, I look again around the bothy loving its warmth and natural feel. This boat-house is seldom used by the family in winter. There is no doubt in my mind that I'll be back again by January. Four months . . . the seriousness of the situation washes over me. I am numb. Whatever the outcome of the next few months, I feel at peace – accepting, but numb too.

The bed is neatly folded away into a daytime couch. I have wrapped and packed glass-wear into drawers along with plates and bowls. There's one treasured coffee mug with blue glaze hand prints of two sweet granddaughters.

Even as I write the labels "Vivien's stuff" to lie on each drawer's contents, I wonder at my doing it. Bedding, towels – everything freshly laundered and packed in plastic along with moth balls – more fastidious attention than usual to the business of being away. As I handle the moth balls I remember the large spider in the sink last night and shudder remembering it emerging from the plug hole. Bent long black legs! Living this close to woodland and being on a coastal strip, brings both joy and the reality of insect life.

Outside, there is no distance to the sea's edge. Overhead are branches from a huge oak and alongside the oak, a bench facing west – facing the sunsets. Think of any seascape picture with grassy banks, add a few sailing boats, iron flat any waves leaving some gentle ripples for the last rays of sun to dance off, and sit quietly for the stillness to penetrate. Learn this recipe and repeat it daily. Now watch the sun sink lower and the horizon grow pink as it rises to meet it, and pinker . . . until the sound of any movement you make seems clumsy amidst such perfection.

Here the sky is unusually vast for England. I sit sometimes alone and sometimes with a friend and always there is magic in those moments; a magic that moves painters to replicate it in water colour. Watery art is in step with delicate scenery in Bushton where water colour artists are plentiful. My friends love to visit and we have conversations that don't happen elsewhere.

The Purple Envelope

I close my suitcase and leave this dwelling behind to drive to my daughter in Kent. I will fly out to South Africa tomorrow.

* * *

Around this time at the University of Pretoria, Clare, who had been Michael's first girlfriend, made an entry in her diary

today, Michael sent me a text.

We haven't spoken in weeks. I'm not sure why, we just didn't. Last time I saw Mike, was at Josh's house and he was having a good time with his friends. I felt out of place and uncomfortable, so I left early. After all, I'm only a 'sort of friend' of his now.

Emily had sent me a package from England and Michael dropped it off at my parents. I wonder if he still sees me sitting on the wall, waiting for him to come and visit me when he stops at their gate . . . I wonder if he ever goes in, if he imagines me in the kitchen making him his favourite lemon drink the way I see him when I go there . . . . I wonder if he still sets the time on the digital clock in the kitchen that keeps going out because somebody always unplugs it . . . no, no, now is not the time, now I have to tell about the text . . . so, Mike went to drop my package and my mom phoned me to say he is looking ill, thin, tired. I phoned him yesterday, and he said he was going to the doctor today, but sure it was nothing. then the text today . . . "it's cancer. Dr says one chemo, if no go then game over"

I closed my eyes; maybe I could pretend for another minute, reality threatens to overwhelm me. tears fall, I don't even try to stop them . . . suddenly I felt very small, very lost. I loved Michael, after all that has happened, I loved him, with my whole heart, my very being and it scared me beyond imagination to think that I may lose him, that he may die, that things may never get better for us . . . . I felt my heart leak out under my closed lids.

Annette found me like that, curled up on my room's hard carpet . . . I couldn't tell her, only showed her the text, I was clutching the phone to my breaking heart. She understood, she knew how many dreams were threatened by that one word . . .

* * *

I drive north towards London. The crisply fresh coastal and rural air fades as I enter the outer fringe of London's Home Counties. The small Kentish town where Emily lives is farming country, but is within London's commuter belt. It's easy to get to the airport from there. My flight is booked for Friday – the following day.

At her home I have a call with Michael's father in South Africa. We are not together and he, living at some distance but not too far from Michael, has made his way to see him.

"What's he eating?" I ask.

"Oh you know what they eat," I am told.

The activities of these young men didn't always leave time for home cooking. Takeaways, chips, and who knows what else, filled emergency food-stops between the meals that they cooked.

"Get in some fresh fruit and especially fresh vegetables," I say.

"Find pineapple for him," I go on.

Where did that idea come from!

"It must be fresh pineapple," I insist, wondering why I say it. What do I know!

Later I hear from David that a box of fresh produce is there – on the counter for when I get back.

"He needs it now," I say across six thousand miles.

"Make sure he has the pineapple."

With Emily and her young family, together we anticipate what is to come. I have never encountered cancer. I am fairly blissfully ignorant.

Emily is finding out how to make a healthy difference with environmental changes, such as, which type of pans to use in the kitchen, and shopping for organic produce. Tanya is discovering foodstuffs that are rich in the wonder cancer fighter vitamin B17, like apricot kernels. She has bought some already.

That was the first I heard of a list, that was to grow very long, of aids to overcome cancer. Excellent if the cancer hasn't got a grip; if it's been caught early. Those are the two elements of the disease that make any approach to combat it, easier.

Take preventative measures; catch it early and nip it in the bud.

The situation is serious but I have peace about whatever the outcome of the next few months is to be. My flight leaves the next day.

Chicken Soup for the Soul would have made good travel reading for that flight home.

I arrive in Johannesburg on 1st September – the first day of spring in South Africa.

4

> Don't believe what your eyes are telling you,
> All they show is limitation.
> Look with your understanding.
> Jonathan Livingston Seagull

In Johannesburg the air is dry and brown fields are a contrast to England's summer green. Nowhere is that more clear to see than as you come in to land at Johannesburg airport where hopes are high that spring rain will soon break winter's drought. Britain's lush green is still imprinted in my mind, and imprinted with it, the view from the bothy where trees mark the near horizon, and cold sea the far distant horizon.

Passport control has a slow moving queue, but at last, with my baggage and customs behind me, I look for him . . . and happily see that both of my sons are there.

Michael has a goatee beard. It's a trend, but even a full beard wouldn't have hidden from me that pale face which is a face of pain. We hug but there's otherwise no easy response to my arrival.

Why so strained? He is sorry to have interrupted my plans for a trip to Canada. It will be cancelled without a thought.

It's good to be with my two sons. We talk and relax as Anthony drives us from the airport. We start thinking through the several ideas that Michael's caring and creative siblings have for us.

I'm told how Gaby, the daughter of an old friend, has offered her help – has hi-tech equipment and will work with his vibrations for a different picture of what's going on in his body. Knowing nothing, I question little the authoritative tone of friends who care and who know something.

There's good reason to use time wisely with cancer, especially one like this which is so far developed, and so we waste no time and arrive at Gaby's consulting room at noon that day. Gaby is stunning with too many natural red glints in her buzz of hair to say it is mid-brown. Blue eyes reflect light – almost phosphorescent it's not easy to meet the brightness of their gaze. We talk awhile and Michael settles down.

In the waiting room tiredness overwhelms me. There were too many disturbances on the night flight, and too little space to be comfortable, so with heavy eye lids and dull mind I'm soon dozing.

I remember my friend in Cape Town some ten years earlier, phoning me to ask if I would bake and deliver a surprise chocolate cake to Gaby for her fortieth birthday. I remember making the cake and being questioned at home, "why are you doing this?"

I hadn't considered why.

I would do it for my far away friend and for her brave daughter who had been through a lot. And so it was that she had the cake.

"It's from your mother," I said.

She held it with appreciation and closed the door.

Now here she is giving us her time and expertise. We later receive a lengthy report on her findings.

Back at home, I find a card from a teacher at Michael's old school. She recommends a second opinion from her friend a surgeon. We see him on Monday . . . a wise caring man. He looks at the x-rays and agrees with the oncologist. Surgery would be impossible.

This man has charisma. He speaks quietly. His stillness is deafening. I want him to breathe and play with papers – or his pen. Why doesn't he move – make a call. He's speaking again . . . he had heard about Michael from the school teacher, she had told him about Michael as a pupil, how she remembered him.

"Here is my private number. Please call me at any time . . . 2o'çlock in the morning isn't a problem." He said it so very kindly.

It's our move and we're rooted to our chairs. He hands us the x-rays now back in their envelope, and somehow I'm freed from my paralysis. We leave and it seems there's no progress, but there is a growing acceptance of reality.

The list of experts is growing. Friends pass their details on to us, urging us that their contact must be seen.

The homeopath, skilled in natural health methods, was once a medical doctor and had experience in Mexico in a cancer research centre. He needs only one x-ray to get the picture but he goes through them all. He sees the large germ cell cancer and sees the many cannonballs – baby cancers in the lungs – metastases or secondary cancers. I know the words now, know the response each word gets from people who Know. That primary tumour is hard and filling the spaces in the rib cage between the lungs, stomach, heart and kidneys. Of great concern are the 'cannonballs' in the lungs.

This isn't like the childhood tonsillitis or scarlet fever that the homeopath treated in Michael before. In his face, in his eyes, it seems he is not finding words to bring together the conclusion he's drawn from the x-rays – to speak it into the silence of the room. His head moves from side to side so slightly as to be almost imperceptible and he reiterates the principle changes in diet that he's already talked about – and yes, chemotherapy. His eyes follow us as we leave the consulting room. In them is deep concern.

"YOU MUST SEE THE HERBALIST,' said another friend into my ear through the telephone piece. She urged it saying her friend had not lost her hair and had lived for six more years after taking herbs.

We drove the long difficult distance to find the house where small rooms comprised a waiting room and consulting room. Even arriving there at 8 o'clock we found the room filling up. Heather the herbalist had fitted us into her already full day.

As she talked about her herbs, many imported from around the world, I wondered if it was possible to drink all the herbal tea each day, that she said was necessary, or to eat all the grated raw carrots and beetroot she recommended.

"He can't!" I protested.

"He doesn't like beetroot." It sounded feeble.

"Does he want to live?" she sharply retorted.

Early on I learnt the importance of carotene and vitamin A and about finding non-acidic vitamin C, and about selenium with vitamins A C and E.

Another cancer expert offered a blue liquid preparation at great expense and it may have been the answer if we had taken it. It came with the instruction (among many) to eat broccoli and brown rice every day for the rest of his life, and never again put anything in his mouth that came from a pig.

A feeling of being overwhelmed is growing.

A gift is delivered to us. It's to extract the juice from the fruit and vegetables. How thoughtful of Emily's mother-in-law.

A friend arrives with a supply of purified water for him to drink, bringing with it evidence that there is heavy metal contamination (mercury) in our drinking water.

Another friend sends a book about the vital importance in the healing process, of drinking plenty of water.

Tanya comes with the vitamin B17 capsules that arrived from the States at considerable cost. From her research we learn of some Himalayan people who have unusual longevity. Important in their diet are the fruit and kernels of apricots which are a rich source of this vitamin – otherwise known as laetrile. But even our apple pips and pumpkin seeds contain traces of it and we throw them away. One book that I read called Dead Doctors Don't Lie, taught me still more, including things about the drug industry that were confusing.

And so we all try to eat apricot kernels and pumpkin seeds, and add cinnamon and honey to our diet. We avoid carbonated drinks and stay away from water with heavy metal, and from cigarette smoke, and too much sugar and highly refined foods, as well as artificial preservatives; and we avoid many other things that we are told are suspicious. Some are surprising – unexpected things like excessive electric light in the dark hours – even that which glows into a bedroom from a street lamp.

Committed to fight this from all corners, I read and learn a great deal. Many books are gifts. We learn how to grow bean shoots and learn the value of alfalfa whose tap roots penetrate deep into the ground and reach minerals that so often barely exist at top soil level.

We read how our blood group affects our lives and is part of who we are. From that I understand why the homeopath advised no more meat for Michael for at least ten years, and preferably for the rest of his life . . . that his supply of the enzymes that digest meat may be only marginally sufficient; and I read that, among other things, fresh pineapple can be beneficial for this.

Most of all we understand the value of natural foods and keep an awareness of the shifts in opinion by writers on nutrition.

Michael doesn't complain.

At last I meet the oncologist. The oncology department at our local hospital will become very familiar and today I am relieved that the treatment can get started. Michael introduces me and the doctor responds,

"Your mother . . . ? Not overseas?"

We shake hands.

"I'm back," I smile.

He is nice. He is young and thorough. I am told he's right up to date with the latest information that's available globally from on-going research.

It has been identified as germ cell cancer. Not sarcoma. There are lots of questions and we hear things that prepare us for what is to come.

Some side effects of chemotherapy are sickness, hair loss, weakened mouth and nose membranes, and pins and needles in feet and hands. From a wide range of side effects, there are some slight differences in how people are affected. The doctor recommends and advises about life issues, forewarns that there's a possibility of infertility and suggests where to have sperm frozen and stored. Michael is prepared. They are both new pilots; they like each other.

Chemo will begin on Monday, five days a week for three weeks, and then a break.

The diagnosis was a week earlier. I wonder about even a day's delay. In my mind's eye, I see something like cauliflower florets swelling in the connective tissue between his organs. It grows rapidly and painlessly in his chest cavity – baby cancer balls in his lungs. What do I know? I know Monday is five days away and this huge growth probably took between four and six months to grow. We will learn to take it one day at a time. There are many unknowns in the days and possibly months ahead.

And among the unknowns, we will meet a new side to people we know.

Among them are some colleagues at Michael's place of work.

Early on I came home to a phone message from a company director. It went something like this,

"Hello Michael, I called because we have heard the news which has shocked and dismayed us. We are very sorry and want you to do whatever is necessary for your recovery. Don't worry about your job, it is here and when you can be at your desk we will be pleased to see you. We want to see you get better. Be sure to take care of what you need first." The last words were said with emphasis. I listened to it again, touched by his understanding, and his care for Michael's needs.

With medical decisions made, we face the future with some inevitability. With the start of chemotherapy a new challenge begins and we are on starter blocks. Speed isn't the quest, combat is.

5

> It sometimes seems our troubles
> and the days and hours that contain them
> overshadow those moments of stillness
> where the quiet rings with peace.
> Mike Koehler

Michael is ready for chemotherapy and on Monday 10th September we are introduced to a procedure that will become a familiar routine. A cocktail mix of chemicals drips into his arm for most of the morning. A blood sample for testing is taken prior to its commencement and it shows that his human Chorionic Gonadotropin (HCG) count is 311,000. In a healthy man the HCG count is between zero and five. In a woman, it's a hormone that is produced during pregnancy.

For four hours chemicals are administered that should selectively kill cells which are cancerous, while not being a threat to healthy cells, other than to temporarily damage his hair, gums and stomach lining. I hear the mention of chemical names which make up the cocktails. I know the word platinum but the others are foreign sounding to me.

The Purple Envelope

We return the next day. It is Tuesday 11th September 2001, a day that is remembered as a day of tragedy. We watch TV seeing the assault on the World Trade Centre Twin Towers in New York. That aggressive assault that caused irreversible changes and such great heartache and we watch the amateur video shown on TV with unbelief.

The world mourned the loss of human life and we mourned for them too while embracing our own tragedy. The events of 9/11 shocked us – those people had no fighting chance.

It is the obvious that occurs to us. Death is a singular and personal experience and for those left behind there is the inescapable sense of loss. Whether the loss is of a son overcome in battle, or overcome by illness or an accident, there is a feeling of loss. Whether it is in China, New Zealand, or Washington; no matter the skin colour, or home language; whether the victim has achieved greatly, or is uneducated, people experience their own sense of loss. The world grieved for wasted life in New York on 9/11. That loss for victims' loved ones involves deep sorrow.

Daily Michael subjects himself to a long attack by poisons targeting some of his cells. The poisons course through his veins, lethal to his cancer cells while causing minor damage to some others. These others are vulnerable because like cancerous cells, they divide rapidly, but unlike cancer cells their growth is not out of control. The treatment is giving him a chance to live.

It's day three and we know the routine. Sitting with the needles and plastic pouches of potent chemicals for the better part of four hours gives one time to think and consider and always watch the activities of two bright accommodating, positive young nurses. It seems that it's largely due to them that the outpatients at the local oncology centre, has a cheerful mood.

Patients seated in comfy leatherette reclining chairs all have questions and they get answers from the nursing sisters Marie and Gill. Attention is on the benefits and probabilities of the process for cure, and less on difficulties, although the patients are listened to and heard with empathy.

To that "why me?" question, we hear that everyone is born with the potential for cancer. We have these alien cells forming from time to time in our healthy bodies. It's just another of the fights that go on internally, which we aren't aware of while it's happening. Our immune systems deal with overcoming them.

Visitors and patients submit to the experienced skill of the medical team. Their light competent mood prevails.

"Take what comes" says Michael.

He is among the fortunate ones whose medical insurance will cover the costs.

Many of the patients and their loved ones are bravely chirpy too. It seems that my own resources are depleted. Deep down there is a sense of gratitude for them and the doctors, but I'm not one of the brave ones who present a bright exterior. I drink in all that is going on – and drink the filter coffee whose aroma welcomes us each morning. The TV is usually tuned for the sports channel.

In the evening of that third day Clare visited him at home and they chatted for hours. She was in her first year of training to be a nurse. She brought extra information from the university to add to answers we already had to our many questions. Later she chose oncology as the career direction to take.

On that Wednesday night it turned unexpectedly cold. Winter in Johannesburg is often sunny and pleasant and is usually warm during the middle hours of the day. September temperatures can drop surprisingly low – it is part of Johannesburg's high altitude weather changes that we are used to.

That night Michael woke me at one o'clock. He couldn't breathe. He coughed but his lungs were not responding. I called Dr Mac and later at his rooms, Michael stumbled along, bent over and walking slowly. Pneumonia was diagnosed. He was admitted to hospital. The sudden cold had been enough to trigger this infection because his immune system was weak.

He shared the ward with Ted, a man who was back for chemotherapy after a long period in remission. Their conversation was good for Michael and I found myself saying a quiet word of thanks on his behalf. From then on the boxed fruit juice, from Ted's fruit juicing company, has been the one I buy at the supermarket, and Ted will never know it.

The pneumonia caused little interruption in the cancer treatment. Anti-biotics were intravenously administered along with chemicals.

Friends surround his bed. Some weep quietly in my presence, but not in his. Some of those friends had been in school with him from age three.

Clare wrote in her diary:

I had my 'house formal' while Michael was ill, but he was doing ok, so I went. I would have wanted him to go with me, but, having learned my lesson the last time, I didn't even ask. I wore my matric farewell dress, like all the other 1st year students. My hair was pinned back and had blue colouring on the tips, I loved it! The evening wasn't as much fun as I hoped it would be and I thought about Michael a lot. We have been seeing a lot more of each other and I was really enjoying having him back in my life.

The next time I phoned him he didn't answer. Instead he sent me a text (he seems to have really mastered the skill of giving bad news by text) to say he was admitted to hospital and it may be a Pulmonary Embolism. So, I rushed over there . . ., my heart stopped as I walked into the room, he looked so pale and ill and thin. I slowly, quietly walked over to him. His eyes were closed but even then, I could see they were sunken with deep dark circles. He had a face mask on giving him oxygen, I wanted to kiss him, but his lips were a horrible blue colour and I was too scared to take off the mask, so I sat down next to him and took his hand. Without opening his eyes he laced his fingers through mine and gripped my hand. We sat like that for a long time, him struggling to breathe and me listening to every sound he made. Slowly he opened his eyes; I was relieved that they were still the same blue colour. I don't know why I thought they would have changed . . . he seemed so different. I was happy to see the soul I loved was still in there.

He stared at me, finally saying "what have you done with your hair?" and I had to smile.

September comes and goes. October . . . and the routine towards combating cancer continues . . . Michael has visitors at home. Doug, loud, alert with so much laughter – Josh, quiet, caring, clever. Rugby playing Dion is sensitive;

loud, boisterous funny Colin; lovely Clare who's so young; Sarah striking and set for success; Fiona silent in her gentle sensitivity.

From his friends at church there are daily visits. Elders and the minister come and pray at his bedside. The young people who remembered Michael in their Friday fun evenings collected pocket money for a gift, and delivered it to his bedside – plants in a pot that was moulded to resemble a lion's head.

A friend from church turned to him and tears welled up as she said,

"I am so sorry".

"Don't worry," he said quietly, "It's fine."

* * *

It was later, months later, that I realized I had been protected from reality – a reality that the people at church were aware of.

What I learned from a lady there, was that the numbers in a regular Bible study group swelled from the usual twelve people to sixty in the week when his diagnosis came through. After Wednesday's discovery of cancer, news went around quickly and Thursday's study became a prayer meeting. A newcomer, who had not met Michael, wondered how this could be as he heard the prayers, some with tears, and as he heard how the people talked about him. I found this out by chance when I called at a book shop in a nearby town, and met his wife Barbara.

She said her husband spoke in a surprising way about the evening and the response that his illness evoked in those Christians. From that day on they both included Michael in their prayers, as others did.

In that prayer group there were students, accountants and IT people. A truck driver, an insurance broker, and a banker too, and with them ministers, domestic workers and housewives as well as salesmen and others. They were of several different racial groups, and both the unemployed and multi millionaires were represented.

I was driving to Emily's from the bothy on that day, not knowing, as Michael did, that he may not live to see Christmas.

But I had been aware of something on the day after my return from England. It was Sunday. As I walked into the church building, and before I had even taken my seat towards the back, I was aware of something I could not identify. So if not identifiable, how can I write of it . . . of the sense of angelic presence in the air. A lightness – an out of this world lightness. How good and unspeakable it was.

I took my seat. The service proceeded. I was home with people who had new reason to love one another.

I see love differently now. Love is shown in many ways, some practical, some tender empathetic ways. Sometimes it involves sacrifice but that's incidental as the giver of love doesn't count the cost because that has less importance than the gift whether it's time or help or comfort. Through touch, words and provision, the love gift is delivered. I recognize it daily, and yes, I was at home with people who had reason to love each other more.

Michael's cousin Sarah is in her gap year in England. He receives this from her.

"I am currently in the process of organizing a flight over to visit you. Stephen has been very kind and helpful and is trying to organize a cheaper flight deal, which depends on flight availability. We also hope that flights will be running due to the terrible happenings in New York and Washington. I really hope that the trip is able to go ahead as I am very much looking forward to seeing you. I have a lot to tell you about . . . . probably three years worth in fact. I hope you have a few days to listen! Hopefully I will not bore you too much . . . lots and lots of love from Sarah and all of the family in England.

6

It's November and treatment continues as before. There's a certain monotony in it. Always the same nurses always groomed and having dropped children at school before arriving at the hospital. Always cheerful and friendly, they make vein finding easy while answering questions. They tend to maybe half a dozen patients and always seem to be on top of what they do so well. The bags of cocktails drip slowly into him and we vainly wonder if he'll be lucky – that his body will respond. Only time will tell. The nausea, the hair loss, the pins and needles are not in the early days.

Three weeks of treatment and a week off continues. During the week off, something of a feeling of wellbeing starts to return and Michael is glad at these times, that he is able to go to work.

Early preparations are being made for Christmas and a festive office party has been arranged. One of Michael's colleagues comes to the house from time to time and as she leaves this time, she appeals to me.

"Make sure he gets to the party," and then she says, "no, I'll pick him up – but please encourage him to be there."

She turns to leave, but there's something I want to ask.

"He has had extraordinary care from you all. I mean, the freedom to come and go in the office without fear of losing his job still goes on and they are true to their promise even now that it's been months."

"Vivien, he has earned it. In their eyes he earned it right back when he first came . . . perhaps you don't know about that?"

My mind goes back to that first day. It's not what she was talking about, but I think of him leaving the house on the first morning.

"Good luck son."

"Yeah, thanks Mom."

For a moment I thought that I should say no more, but on I ploughed . . .

"When you get there," I hesitated knowing I was doing a mother thing and willing myself to stop right there . . . but on I went, "when you get there, the first person you're likely to see, is the receptionist. She has a name and she has a life."

"Yes," he nodded thoughtfully.

Encouraged, I went on,

"There's likely to be a mid-morning break when someone will see that you get drinks – a tea boy, or girl. That person has a name and a life. It's good to know that."

Michael left for work and left me to chores.

Doreen is talking.

"Vivien, he'd had six months experience when he joined the company at nineteen years of age. He was given maintenance and routine stuff to do. Back then, the company had a problem with compatibility. It was a major project for a government department and they couldn't link up. Even the experts they brought in were no help. Michael wasn't involved with it at all, but he overheard discussions around him and asked a couple of questions. One evening he stayed behind for three or four hours and presented the solution in the morning. They vowed to take him seriously right then and have never forgotten."

How well I know of his curiosity which so often fed his love for a challenge. Doreen's story reminds me of many challenges.

I thought back to when I met his geography teacher at a school open day. Her experience with him, she told me, was that he listened. I was not impressed. There is surely nothing out of the ordinary in that?

"He was fully present in the class," she said. "His input was on track and it stirred interest which sometimes led to a chat forum, and I would enjoy my subject more."

Yes, he thought about what he heard, and his curiosity came into play. It sort of fed him and the people around him.

Looking back I remember that, perhaps more than anything, I wanted my children to find their niche in life. I discovered that it is often the contribution not the project that matters. It is in involvement and relationships that realization of many things comes.

It was in 1981 that like his brother and sister, Michael was born three weeks later than his due date. A late arrival had been right for the other two babies. Emily and Anthony who were then ten and eight were born after 43 weeks as well. But I was older for this pregnancy, and that was of concern to some doctors. I was well and happy that a third child was on the way. He would enjoy his childhood like the others who could play out with friends in the safe suburb where we lived. They were good days in the Cape in South Africa where you could rely on warm summer sunshine.

We decided to let biology determine the birth date. We did so after hearing the opinion of an experienced midwife and two doctors who placed more than usual emphasis on natural birth.

And so it was that he was born early one Sunday morning – this so called laat lambetjie (late addition to the family). A caesarean section became necessary and while I was still in an anaesthetized state, the gynaecologist spoke clearly into my ear,

"You have a beautiful big baby boy."

In those days we more often found out at birth what our baby's gender was. In my unconscious state I knew all was well.

I slept on and later woke in a ward to see nurses hurrying around. Finally they brought a baby that was clearly not mine – well it was clear to me.

"No, that isn't my baby!"

Another baby was brought, and that one was not mine.

"Please bring my baby."

When he came I knew without looking at the tag on his arm that this was whom I had carried for nearly ten months as surely as if I had seen him before. The bond was already made with this big beautiful barrel-chested baby boy who had curly blond hair. He was strong. We were in tune.

Seven days later the mild jaundice was clear and we were at home where family life began for this brand new person who was loved from the start by his father, sister and brother, and who always would be loved.

He was three months old when we sat with friends to see the royal wedding of Prince Charles and Lady Diana Spencer on television. There was some awe attached to that day in South Africa, once part of the British Commonwealth. There were Union Jacks, pots of tea, mugs of beer and other British symbols. Resident Americans joined us too. Michael was doing well. His growth chart was as good as it gets. He was a good natured baby and he seemed, even then, to love life.

It is twenty years on, December of 2001, and our hope is that twenty years isn't all that he'll have. Four months is a long time with daily pain and discomfort, and debilitating tiredness. I left England anticipating that he would be over this by now. The work and temporary home that I left behind, as well as the people whom I cared for, all seemed light years away.

Cousin Sarah came from England, making it part of her gap year travels; and so did Emily and her family. Their visits were wonderful for us.

In her diary Clare wrote:

Emily, Stephen and the boys came over from England. It was so good to see them. Emily and I have remained rather close over the last year or so – ever since I visited them in England. I went to church with Michael. I stopped going to church sometime during the year and it felt strange to be back, but I loved standing next to this tall, although much thinner, balding man. I've always admired Michael's faith, so blind, so totally devout, I envied him . . .

Around that time, as Christmas approached, Clare wrote,

Something Michael said:
The day Michael said he is tired and he wants this all to end was the scariest, saddest day. I so desperately wanted him to WANT to live, to WANT to fight, but, the colour had left his eyes and in that moment I thought he wanted to die.

7

> Whoever you are,
> with eyes that have forgotten how to see,
> from viewing things already too well-known,
> take another look around you.
> Ranier Maria Rilke

Everyone knew in August that without a huge fight Michael wouldn't see Christmas.

And now it's that time of year. There's tinsel and coloured lights; a tree decorated with festive golden bells, stars and baubles. There's fun in the air and we live vicariously through the children, because it's Christmas.

Barry the cat lurks furtively, positioning himself under low branches of the tree. He keeps Anthony in view, waiting . . . the temptation is strong for forepaws to playfully biff dangling tree trinkets, boxer style. Anthony unwisely glances away and Barry's game begins, and lasts for two seconds before Anthony is on to it. Jingling Xmas bells fall from the tree. Barry flees using a well used escape down the passage and through the open bathroom window.

Anthony races outside to confront him as he comes through the window. It's been played before. Anthony's girls giggle and roll their eyes as their Dad sports with his favourite pet.

There's respect for speed and intelligence between man and cat. Wrapped and ribboned gifts are colourfully heaped around the tree. It entices kids' as well as cats' curiosity.

It's a southern hemisphere mid-summer Christmas and the day runs on in a long established Jones way. For us this year, the difference is that we are together. All of us together and for me, the excitement in the children's faces seems to glow brighter than any festive decoration.

Emily and her family arrived in South Africa from England, a journey of no less than six thousand miles. They will see Mike knowing that nothing about his future is certain, indeed he may not have one. But that he is with us is the best gift we have for Christmas. We live for the day we have. It's all we know that we have.

We find that the cousins have a great affinity for each other, and real attachment for their seldom seen aunts and uncles. The kids have little if any memory of these people.

Three years apart is a lifetime for small children. It's time we relish – but among us, there are two who eye each other cautiously.

I had guessed that Emily would not share her brother Anthony easily, and Tanya, this woman who is his wife, had wept sadly with her, for Michael. Their mutual edginess is blunted today by their concern for him.

Michael is quiet. He sits aside from us with arms leaning on thighs holding the burden of his upper body. His once heavy hair is thin and tufty.

"Be careful what you wish for," his friend chides, remembering the former complaints about his hard-to-handle mane of hair before chemotherapy.

Today there's a shade of warmth in his expression which is otherwise placid. His girlfriend sits with her arm loosely linked in his. Her hand softly rests on his thigh. With mutual stillness they look across at the activity. She is in tune with his low energy level.

There are no surprises in the annually repeated events of a Jones Christmas day, but Michael this year eats less than the little that's on his plate, and then he slips away to another room to sleep. It's a three hour sleep.

Cousins and siblings drink grape juice from wine glasses at the children's own table. Their table, like ours, has Tanya's usual touch. Once a florist she snips what looks, to the casual onlooker, like a random bunch of flowers from the garden and drops them into a vase where they fall into a perfect arrangement.

How does she do that every time!

The pudding is aflame with brandy. It's festive and so we agree to a small portion. We each eat richly from the hot fruit pudding. Brandy butter melts in slow motion over it. A silver coin may be in our portion – competition is high for this lucky find. It's our kind of fun.

Lots of effort goes into pulling the crackers and plastic nonsense gifts roll onto the floor where a child will retrieve it laughing and claiming it against protests from the table. Whistles and spinning tops . . . We smile at corny jokes because everything's easy. Paper hats are put on for only a moment before being tossed aside.

Mike sleeps.

Afterwards, we sit around languidly until Anthony rouses us for French cricket. Will the ladies prefer croquet? We join in with cricket, thankful not to risk the tricky grass sods on this lawn deflecting our mallet shots which frustrate and embarrass us.

"Oh, Gran," they laughingly commiserated last year, glad that their luck was in and I filled the loser spot.

Michael is with us. Again he leans forward in his chair. Cricket is his game. He watches, and he and Clare look with equal stillness across at the activity in the pool. The children race to the pool, and are soon swimming or riding astride inflated rubber sharks.

Anthony teases playfully and Kevin goofs around with the kids – both being kids again themselves.

Michael is weak, and this is hard for him to endure. Surrounded by loved ones attuned to his state, he soaks up a love aura as he has all day, seeing the children laughing at the uncles' antics and teases.

Mike and Clare sit in their own private reverie. He is alive. We are complete and each of us grows; each of us knows a new level of appreciation. Bonds are strengthened.

Life's values shift because the reality is that death may be lurking nearby.

Before leaving to go home, we group ourselves with our backs to the high hedge for the obligatory family photo. The camera timer takes a while to set up . . . too long a stretch for Michael to remain standing. When the picture is developed, the print will show him crouched on haunches. Two year old Aden beside him finds that he's at his eye level. He is pictured nestled against him with a child's tenderness.

* * *

This is the Christmas day entry that Clare made in her diary:

Then came Christmas
    . . . it's at Anthony and Tanya's. The kids are all playing and the adults talking nonstop. I can feel Michael's exhaustion, he hardly speaks and will only nod in reply to whatever anyone asks, but he smiles often and I can see he is enjoying this, even when he can't stay awake any longer. So often these days, I feel him leaving me to go off somewhere in his own world, I try to follow but he won't let me. It scares me. In one of those moments, when he is off somewhere, I sneak a sideways look at him. He is so so thin, his skin almost translucent, his wonderfully thick hair has fallen out in patches and there are circles under his eyes. My heart aches. I know he is one of a kind. I'll never know anyone like him again and it breaks my heart to think of the cruelty of someone so absolutely wonderful dying too young. I look away, I don't want him to know what I thought, but as I turn he squeezes my hand and I know I have been caught.

* * *

I've noticed that Michael is seeing more of Clare lately and is usually in a cheerful mood afterwards. They are friends.

But it wasn't to last.

Later (it was years later) Clare and I met up again. As we chatted, Clare told me,

"I can't remember how it started and I'm not sure how it ended. I went to a new year's party with Michael and in my diary I wrote,"

We had such fun, the way we always do, but something has changed between us. In the last few months many things have been said that should have been kept quiet.

Clare continued, "he had come to visit me at university and we ended up having a huge argument because I wanted him to eat the healthy things he was supposed to and he didn't want me to tell him what to do. I was unsure of what to say to him, he seemed uncharacteristically edgy and snappy. I was scared that he would leave me, so I was unreasonable and started arguments with him for no reason so that there would be a reason why he left . . ."

She paused, thinking back to those events, and went on, "we had a massive argument. I don't know about what any more, but it ended with me getting out of his car and walking in to my parent's house, not looking back and waving and waving again as I always did, just going in and closing the door and not speaking to him again for many many months.

"Oh, we talked about it later, but we seemed to recall what happened very differently. As they say, 'there is your story, my story and the true story'.

"Emily kept me updated with how he was and he was so often in my thoughts and prayers. How young I was then, how little I understood of life and love . . ."

* * *

Into the New Year, blood tests show that the blood count is down to 27 on its way to zero from the original 311,000. He's had four months of treatment – two different cocktails, and we are preparing for more chemotherapy.

At home I sit at a table waiting for my friend Pat to answer the phone. Pat has struggles that would floor me, and I keep in touch with her. The ringing tone continues as I wait for her to pick up, and while waiting, my finger toys with the fine pages of a book lying there.

The finger traces words embossed on the leather cover and I wonder why a Bible is there.

Who left it?

The phone continues to ring unanswered. I flick the book open and my gaze falls on strong words on the open page of Philippians.

It reads, "For indeed he was sick almost to death: but God had compassion on him, and not only on him but on me also, least I should have sorrow upon sorrow."

I hang up not leaving a message, but I will never again doubt that he will regain his life fully. I will no longer wonder. From now on, I'll just wait.

Philippians 2v27

8

'The challenge is to exist fully and love fully in the series of moments that go together to form today. In this way, the truly important things, your real priorities, show themselves to you.'
Burton A. Presberg

Our commitment to find alternative foods that would nourish if he only absorbed a little, continues, but as time goes on my expectations about diet change. I listen to Michael. He seems to know instinctively what he needs and it seems important that he has confidence. So when he says "I won't be able to eat," or simply, "just can't drink it," I listen.

Sometimes he nods "OK," as I offer carefully prepared food, but then I clear it away later thankful if he has taken just one mouthful or sip. But over and over I clear away untouched food. People talk about my wise food adjustments and I feel a fraud because he doesn't eat much of what I prepare.

We tell the doctor what we are doing, seeking his approval and there it is again – that smile, "it will do no harm, it might help," kindly words from Dr Mac.

He the doctor has the means to help. The chemical cocktails are the weapon in this war. It is a war against the invasion of mutant cells. His strategy is skilful, aiming to overcome the enemy within without weakening the natural body.

But how good it is for me to keep busy. The reading keeps me focused and feeling useful. It keeps me doing what good I can do. From all that I read I think only a little matters, but it mattered one day that I had read how to recognize symptoms of stress in his body soon enough to act quickly. And it matters that my energy has direction for Michael. It matters, I think, for his confidence.

There is so much information available and I have access to a wide range of approaches to healing as well as maintaining a healthy body.

I read about cancer victims and learn about research results that indicate some personality types may be more prone to cancer. Michael falls into the type on several counts, his tendency to hoard – hold on to things – hold things close. I read another opinion – that an easy amiable spirit is common in cancer sufferers. It also suggested that there is one blood group that's most likely to get cancer. And there is a genetic factor. His grandmother who was a smoker died of lung cancer.

An oncology nurse once commented,

"These are nice people, they are good humoured. If you had a roomful of cancer patients there'd be a party."

She went on, "In this work, we have nice days. We look forward to seeing the patients, even terminal ones and at the end of the day there's a good feeling because of the individuals. However, everyone is born with the potential for cancer."

One of the sustaining elements for me was the communication I had through email. There was correspondence almost daily, especially with my daughter, and with wise Belinda – a friend in America.

Here's a letter I wrote to Emily:

> Dec 29th. Yes things that help me to feel useful help me to feel OK.
>
> I have learned a lot from the internet, books, Doctors and natural health healers about Michael that is to do with his blood type, his lifestyle habits, and some inherited tendencies. When I read something that fits his profile it is as if I am meeting him in the pages of various books. If it can be said that he has a profile for cancer, then he can learn new lifestyle habits which may overcome those cancer tendencies inherent in him. For example cancers in connective tissue may be there because the circulation is inefficient. The cells become starved of oxygen which would feed and clean the cells. Connective tissue cells are where the starvation happens first. The lungs are in second place and from there the heart doesn't get the oxygen it needs because the lungs are not supplying enough. Working at a computer means his chest is folded exacerbating this problem.
>
> Emily, I learnt from books of some things available at health shops, like hawthorn to strengthen his heart and mistletoe to prevent the formation of cancer cells and improve circulation.

We've found a product which has a unique way of oxygenating and feeding the body at cellular level. There's more Emily but this is to give you the idea.

Friendship has been wonderfully supportive from church. Tonight I'm happy that we are going to the Kings for dinner just as Michael is so much better and is managing food well. All for now, but I will keep in touch . . .

Dinner with the Kings was wonderful and from the array of vegetable dishes Michael ate well. He didn't serve himself from the meats, showing how used he had become to a meat free diet.

Michael preferred to be working on the days when he was not at the hospital but if at the end of a course of chemotherapy it was too much, he stayed at home and rested. Going to the office at nine became a pattern. Sometimes he was told,

"Go home Michael you look tired."

True to their promise they supported the care he needed. It was the energy level that kept him from doing more.

On the days at home we filled some time by watching daytime TV and on many of those dull quiet days I'd observe his attention caught by an advertisement for body lotion which had background music of an unusual quality. It wasn't what he saw in the advert but what he heard, that caused the reaction.

"That music, what is it?" he asked.

The melody was familiar but the arrangement confused us with its electronic hum.

I took on the quest to find that music because there seemed to be healing in it. It was a tricky search and I was ready to give up but made one last call to the body cream company's advertising agents. I had the time to wait for the right person to be located in the company, time to wait for her to return from a conference across the world; time to be patient; time to find geniality in the colleagues taking my calls in her office.

And then quite quickly the right person called me. She kindly offered us a disc copy of their arrangement of Beethoven's Pathetique. Within a few days we had it at home.

There are people out there who resemble angels. They go out of their way, for no reason of gain, to do some kindness that is in their power.

Sometimes a home movie might fill the hours when Michael was too weak to be at the office. A favourite was "O Brother Where Art Thou?" It amused him more with each of many viewings and he would ache from laughing. Hours afterwards I heard his chuckle from somewhere in the house as he recalled a sequence from the movie . . . and I watched too, loving the fun of it.

Friends continued to visit. That affirmation from seven friends from his school days mattered. The mother of one of Michael's school friends was part of a local choir. She talked about him there and he eventually went to talk to them. There was no hype. There was sincerity.

Around that time, his friend Daniel, sadly had a road accident and died . . . and Glen, a local boy his age, got this cancer too and died early. And we still had Michael and we wondered as others did.

He was loved extravagantly through his illness and love was stimulated. People loved and appreciated, from deep within themselves, their own families who were around them. Some went back to church. It could happen to anyone and so it gave new value to their own existence.

When love is stimulated wondrous things that really matter come about, however that love is expressed, and daily it was expressed in many ways.

Whatever else was going on we kept a vision of recovery while living fully in the present happenings.

The cost of Michael's treatment was high but he took disability cover only months before all this started, when he was strong, healthy and only nineteen. It seemed an unusual decision but he made it while under the guidance of a financial adviser that Anthony introduced him to. That decision made a significant difference to managing our expenses.

My trips to England as a companion had previously been a solution to the difficult work situation in Johannesburg and to be in England was no longer a choice for me. The Rear Admiral, Mrs Platt and Mrs Neete in England were a world apart. In reflection, the distance between Johannesburg and the bothy, my abandoned dwelling by the sea, seemed more than mere miles, and so I found temporary employment locally. Grateful in those times for any work in South Africa I accepted a maternity cover in short term insurance. The three months of office work was enough for me. On the last day they asked,

"What will you do now?"

"I am going to write."

9

> When once you have tasted flight,
> you will forever walk the earth with your eyes
> turned skyward, for there you have been,
> and there you will always long to return.
> Leonardo da Vinci

My greetings card for Michael's birthday doesn't go astray this year but others from across the world never reach him.

It meant a lot to me last year that he should get my card in the purple envelope and this year how much it means that he is alive.

It is his 21st this year and we'll go out to dinner. Thankfully he is a week or two away from a course of chemo treatment so he'll manage food. All his friends are invited and we are seated in a private alcove. In the dining room's dim light I see little more than silhouettes – head and shoulder silhouettes of men and girls more often seen under the hospital ward's bright lights. We are all somewhat unable to relax but Michael himself breaks the ice.

Have we become more comfortable seated on the edge of his hospital bed!

Will we ever be the same again? Probably not.

Steve wrote from England, "I usually like to send a birthday card, but you'll understand if I send an email this time . . ."

Like Steve, more people send emails.
Michael's cousin Sarah, on her gap year travels, wrote,

> Everything is seriously amazing and I have just done the first ever bungee created today!! Such a fun experience, chucking yourself off a bridge to be thrown into a river below until your head is totally covered. I did what they call a 'tandem' whereby I dived with someone else (a lad that we travelled with in Oz for a while). Fran didn't fancy it, but I absolutely loved it!
> Saying that, it was not as good as a sky dive in my eyes. We've done two now and they are the most special things ever and give you a sense of freedom, like how you tumble if you fall in dreams.
> We are doing a day trip to the South of New Zealand South Island tomorrow, where we are supposed to see some stunning scenery! It's called Milford Sound and we get to do a cruise along the lake and get a BBQ lunch, luxurious or what!!!!!!
> The money situation is suffering now as there is just SOOOOOO much fun action packed stuff to do here. I don't want to miss out as I'll never get to do some of it again probably.
> For your birthday today . . . a huge kiss and cuddle and have a fantastic day. Thinking of you lots, Sarah xxxx"

And the morning after the birthday, I wrote to Emily

> Mig had a good day for his 21st birthday. The bosses came down to see him and there was champagne in the office . . . on his way home he went to Doug's office as he does sometimes. Back here messages came in and then Chris and Josh arrived and we all went to dinner. We had a great table in an alcove. At home at ten, he and the guys went out again and met Dion and others to play pool. He came home late armed with CDs. He's gone out this morning with Colin to meet others at the Waterside. This afternoon there's a braai for Josh's 22nd and he's seeing some friends this evening. Thank you for the birthday wishes – he's been feeling well, so should enjoy it all. Seeing him in such good spirits has been a good birthday present. Bless you.
>
> Mom Xxxx

A flight in a jet plane is a not-to-be-forgotten experience – an extravagant gift for him from Josh; a twenty minute flight at jet speeds. He blacked out and missed most of the experience. Oh Michael!

He is better to stick with taking his friends around in the microlight. It's in those breaks between chemo courses, when his body recovers enough to be out flying, that we all go up as his passenger.

I am ready for my flight on a day when the wind is right and I wait at the airfield for the essential check that's done prior to any flight. It seems a long wait, but safety depends on its thoroughness.

"Ready for the ride?" He asks. He is ready.

"Mhmm, and no tricks please," I caution.

He gives me an innocent look.

I sit behind him, snugly comfortable. The air where we're going is chilly and I'm well wrapped up in the open cockpit. He has radio communication with air traffic control and knows his way around the north western corner of Johannesburg where there are mountains, the Magaliesburg Mountains. The engine's noise is a clear metallic throb and has been humorously likened to a sewing machine's!

We are down the runway and up . . . yes we are up and I hear Michael's voice through my ear phones. He's asking if I'm alright. As we gain altitude my exposed face feels the chill of the air while body warmth under thermal clothing doesn't change.

"Yes it's great" I shout. I am smiling and he can hear it in my voice.

He tells me we are going down a bit, going to turn, points out things of interest below. I see the tops of trees and nests in them. I see houses with swimming pools, manicured gardens, out of use today, but which are scenes for partying and family gatherings in the warming African sunshine. We spot soft game in a nature reserve – zebras and giraffe, and then he prepares for landing and talks me through everything. I see the runway ahead, a dry brown track running through the African bush and I wait for the bump as we land, but it's little more than a wobble and we come to rest alongside the hanger.

I climb out and walk away from the craft with its vibrations and distinctive fabric and fuel smells. I take off the borrowed protective outer clothing and put aside its rubbery aroma. I remove the earphones and lose the feel of their tough cushions holding my ears, while bringing me sounds of Michael's voice. He would otherwise have been unheard over the noisy engine which was right alongside where we sat. It's stimulating – is a privilege and as we walk back to the hangers we are smiling. What an experience, if an onslaught to our senses.

Our days are full of ups and downs. Between such highlights as flying, there are humdrum happenings – he at the office, and me doing chores and running errands.

At home I deal with some items that his two resident friends left behind, but it is something of an uphill task until the apartment is clear of a 'cloud' that has lingered there. It left along with their books. A collection of empty cola cans, curiously collected and then brought home from Michael's office, is eventually thrown out.

One morning, I engage the gear of my car and drive out of the automated gates that seal off the grounds of our town houses. The road drops away steeply as it skirts the high boundary wall. It's a wall that is topped with electric wiring, installed to protect those of us who live inside from theft, which too often is a violent crime. By the time the road has reached the end of the wall it rises steeply while making a sharp right bend and takes us to the higher ridge. At the intersection, I hesitate only for a moment. The view of the road is open and clearly I may continue on the easy ride to the nearby pharmacist – a place I regularly visit. I have a doctor's prescription, and will buy the canned creamy liquid food called "Ensure" that the pharmacy sells. Its nutritious contents are palatable even for Michael and this, unlike many other foods, is almost never left untouched by him.

So with this purchase, which may be lunch or a snack for Michael today, I walk across the car park, tipping the parking attendant on the way. His presence ensures that my vehicle is not tampered with or stolen while I shop. My fingers make contact with his palm as I press coins there and I feel rough scorched African skin.

Regardless of the preoccupation that is now almost permanently on my mind, I notice that the red post box on the pole is full. It's a small shopping mall, but clearly the business offices and medical consulting rooms generate plenty of correspondence.

The sight reminds me of the birthday card in purple, sent out from an English country village post box, which was never delivered. Was that a lifetime away?

A day or two later, I notice that this box is so full that letters are flapping out.

There is no change the following day and at home I start a string of phone calls to the relevant administrative office managing the postal service, to report that the box was being overlooked. I was passed from one official to another until eventually I spoke to someone who seemed to be the right person to handle the problem.

But the following day the situation remained the same. With each call I made, they took my number but no one called me back. Days later the box was still overflowing and I wondered who was trustingly adding more and more mail to a box that was already jammed so full. The last letters were bent and held in a clamp-like crush in the opening.

I called the office again. This time I was put straight through to Tom who was the right person to speak to. Talking to Tom was congenial. How pleasant to enquire after his health and he mine. Here was the right man and the growing frustration subsided. He, after all, would have an interest in my news and be reasonable. We would sort it out together, I thought, and sure enough we did.

Tom confidently informed me that his man on that route had ridden all around and reported back that there wasn't such a box. Tom could sort it out if I gave him the number on the box. It was another trip to the mall, and another phone call before box number 12, by no means new in the area, was emptied.

From Florida in the States, I hear frustration in an email from Belinda, who has had bad experiences before:

> Hello again Vivien, please let me know Anthony and Tanya's P.O. Box address. I really am cross about this last package not reaching you. There was a carefully made CD with spoken message, pointlessly lost. I found the prettiest note paper in a Hallmark shop. I could not resist sending it to you too, but alas, someone else must have it now! So let's try the Chartres address, o.k.?

I reply,

> I am cross and disappointed too. We talked about it the other day and Anthony and Tanya said they didn't think they had ever lost anything at their P.O. Box. Your kind thought is not overlooked though Belinda.

Her spoken message would have been made especially with Michael in mind – she knew him well, and I pictured the tea cup note-paper guessing she would be feeling as I did a year ago with the lost purple envelope.

Would there forever be postal problems in this wonderful country South Africa, at the southern end of the continent which is sometimes dubbed The Heartbeat of the World.

Regardless of the postal problem, there are a great many messages that do get through.

Michael's cell phone frequently buzzes registering another text message . . .

"A text Michael," I call out, but he's already on it. There must have been thirty today. His friends send many, but plenty are from people further off.

Lots of affirmation in thoughts from young and old. Some say it like this:

'We look forward to seeing you filling the gap in our offices.'

'I miss you every time I walk into the office and your seat is empty. Get well and return to us soon, you are an inspiration to us!!!'

'If positive thoughts are helpful then you have all of mine. May you be flying soon.'

'Hi Jones, be good. Get well soon. We are all waiting for your return. Have a great day.'

'Good luck. Many friends are standing with you – friends like me who really care about you.'

'Behind the grey clouds the sun shines and will soon shine on you.'

And one said: 'Hi there Mike, how are you doing? I'm really sorry that I haven't been writing to you but to tell you the truth I just didn't know what to say?! I'm so glad to hear that you are getting better. I have been praying for you.'

There were those who asked me to convey their thoughts to him and I did because some people don't know – can't find the words to say what they want to say, but have a desire to communicate with him in his pain somehow. There were some who found that it was easier to write their thoughts than to speak to him.

He faces adversity quietly. In his stillness, is he centred and alert for possibilities? In his vulnerability, he has relinquished so much to others.

"Take what comes," he reiterates.

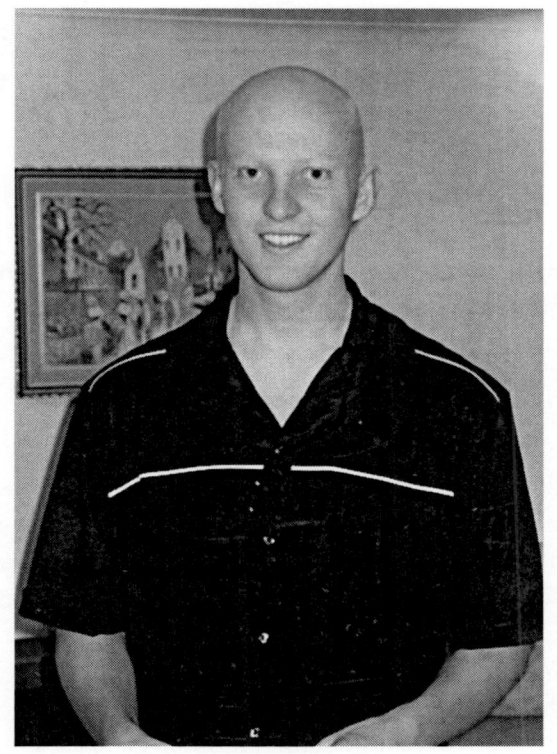

Once again Michael has surfaced in spirit between courses of chemo.

10

*'Life has a way of breaking us,
which means that we can never be the same again.
But God is capable of changing our situation to
such an extent that we can rise above our sorrow.'*
W. Jonker

Once again Michael has surfaced in spirit between courses of chemo. With his humour returning, so does our hope. With health and vigour somewhat returned, and eating not being so much of a problem, the next new course of chemo begins and then health and energy wane again. As each three week course of chemo ends, we wait for the HCG count from blood tests.

He was offered counselling – he shook his head, shrugged his shoulders. It was there if he needed it. A psychologist – himself a cancer survivor – was in the treatment room from time to time, chatting to each of the patients. It was relaxed.

He continues to avoid the early morning traffic crawl through the outer suburbs of Johannesburg, but gets to the office for work each day. Music plays in his car and he has that optimism in his mood.

Michael's baldness turns no heads at a time when men are shaving their heads for that look. But his chemically induced baldness is so perfect that it gets attention and curiosity. It was at the local petrol station where he regularly filled that enduring old vehicle, which was his first car, that the attendant asked,

"How do you do that – perfect baldness without new-growth shadow?" and quickly got Michael's quip,

"Ah well, it's done with chemicals and is very expensive."

He didn't mind the baldness and why would we if he didn't. But losing eyebrows and eyelashes was beyond mere baldness. His weight dropped until at 67kg his 6'2" frame was without much muscle. His appetite was low because of tiredness and taste changes – as well as just being ill. The intake of food was not maintaining his natural body. The drastic weight loss was due in part to the cancer growing process – those alien cells use a supply of nutrients that the body needs; people tell me such things and I listen. What do I know!

The drain of energy that was experienced, worked against his efforts to combat the pressure of the negatives around eating normally. He became a grazer-snacking on bites now and again and the ever ready canned "Ensure" was the most agreeable food that was seldom turned down.

Drinking water helped to keep his mouth moist. He sipped at purified water, often through a straw, knowing that though not easy, it was another positive towards his healing.

Chemotherapy travelling through the blood can reasonably be expected to reach every cell. Most healthy cells are not affected and for those that are, it is temporary.

He would wash his mouth out after meals – sometimes using a topical anaesthetic, but even with only water, the resulting freshness would improve the comfort of those vulnerable and tender gums. A soft tooth brush softened a bit more in hot water was beneficial too. Every little helped towards recovery from this stomatitis – promoting its healing. With a change in balance of organisms too, a yeast infection was a nuisance but was easily treated.

There were some changes to his taste buds. Sweet things in particular became less pleasant to his pallet and while many such taste changes were temporary, this one for sweet things remained. His hands and feet had pins and needles. He had shakes sometimes.

After each full course of VIP (the name given to one of his chemotherapy cocktails) the decline was greater and after this last course he remained inert. I doubt that he was aware that when his body was most burdened, he lay on his back with hands overlapped on his chest. It was several days after chemotherapy that he felt at his lowest. Then his body's production of platelets might have fallen behind – only to catch up days later. In that time the extreme tiredness was debilitating.

With subsequent treatments and the accumulation of toxins, this problem was exacerbated as it takes time for white blood cells to return to normal. We understood that cells already in the blood stream before chemotherapy remain there until they are used or die, but then in the time before the production of blood cells recovered it was hard for Michael to deal with the low energy level. It's the body cells that divide most rapidly, that are most vulnerable to the toxic chemicals.

There were three times that he received blood transfusions. The effect of a blood transfusion was instantaneous. The surge of energy was once most noted as he managed a flight of stairs without stumbling.

"Thank you so very much." My thought is to a man I'll call Jerry who donated the litre of blood. He's one of many people who care and who anonymously, behind the scenes, assist unknown others. Thank you, thank you, thank you to all blood donors and stem cells donors. I am less inclined to complain about anything. My interest in world news is over-shadowed by the news that is in daily living. The appreciation for all blood donors is so very sincere.

Support from individuals that are our close friends is constant.

Local people talk with kindness.

"Michael will be alright," I'm told.

"He thinks positively." It's something many people have said.

I smile, warmed by their positivity. How do they know?

It is their perception.

I do not know how he thinks as he lies on his bed or couch with eyes closed and hands folded over his chest.

I only know gratitude, because close friends care . . . and I smile . . .

At the times when he is back in hospital, visiting hour is often an entertainment. Visitors might include family, church members and local neighbourhood friends.

One typical evening the ex-school friends arrive. It's a year in which some of these young men and young women find their life partners.

Six of them sat at the bed's end and along the sides.
"Hi Mike, how's it?"
"How are you doing?"
Typically he smiles and nods. It's a response.

They sit and pass on current local news; their news. They relate sports events, and dating. They talk about music – and about the boy band from their school that's getting well known. They mention what happens at work – the work they do, and what else they do, and all done with boisterous fun. Michael is propped up against a pile of hospital pillows, crisp white with blue stripes carrying the hospital's name. They re-set the sliding pile of pillows without a break in the conversation. They are loud – well Doug is loud – and funny. The girls watch, and Tanya is there. Her place is always at the end of the bed.

From there she sees Michael's pallor becoming green.
"I'm going to vomit . . ."

Mid-sentence, Josh reaches for the vomit pan and passes it to him. There is no particular attention given to his use of it. They're hearing the build-up of a story, and Michael listens as well, waiting for the punch line. Josh takes the used vomit bowl and with no fuss or comment, it's passed on to a nurse and the unpleasantness isn't registered. The boisterous banter is where they keep their attention. There is so much hospital to dwell on and they give him little chance for it. Set-backs are often given scant attention. It's how they are.

Always after a course of chemotherapy we waited for the HCG results. The original enormous count of 311,000 dropped first to 400 and over the months from there to 27 and down to 4. At 4, it seemed that the doctor's shoulders drooped as he read the results showing that it hadn't reached zero. Was it disappointment being signalled by that body language across to where we watched, before he turned and told us the news.

We went for another opinion; another hospital, another waiting room, another well regarded doctor. She said without hesitation, high dose chemotherapy was necessary.

Dr Mac said the same.

I want to fight his fight with him, maybe I want to fight it for him but I have to leave it. It is his fight. I need to wait and watch and make him as comfortable as he can be – just be there . . . and be available.

He lies in bed inert.

I close in to hug him "I love you very much."

"I know . . ."

. . . it's a murmur; hardly audible.

I happened to be in the room one day when he began to shudder and shake. With a quick response from doctors he was peacefully resting again. Maybe at those low levels I hurt most for him. You see a drawn out illness is hard to endure. In those latter days of chemotherapy I saw him overwhelmed by the process and I wondered how he endured. I felt deep gratitude that he did, and I would sometimes remember the gift that his life had been and thought that if twenty years was all we were to have, then I would find it in me to believe that was how it was to be. I felt wholly and completely at peace. And from those moments of sadness I would return to the battle for his survival.

11

> Each friend represents a world in us, a world
> possibly not born until they arrive, and it is only
> by this meeting that a new world is born.
> Anais Nin

Letters arrived from England, from children in the family and many others who seldom had reason or inclination to write. They wrote about their pets, their school and their sports, and some showed great feeling in telling Michael to get well soon.

The pitch of the messages that reached us, told him that they still saw his worth and value while in the process of fighting for wellness. Who can guess how his progress was influenced by this. I only know that he did go on finding the strength to live and the strength to manage the discomfort.

From an unknown friend,

> "You don't know me but I heard from your friends . . . so sorry to hear about your illness I pray for strength and healing for you at this difficult

time. May these words encourage you in the difficult time you are facing."

Two very young girls in Tampa, who heard about him from Belinda, wrote caring letters.
A local man wrote,
"Hope this rotten business passes soon, and hope this week will be 100% better than last week. Look after yourself. We love you and look forward to seeing you recover and getting back to the things you love to do."

From a friend in England,
"I am looking forward to seeing you shortly and have my fingers crossed that your treatment is very successful. I am sure that it will be. I am sure that you are in good capable hands and that they will do all they can to help you. I am aware of just how emotional the process may well be.

And another wrote,

"We've been wanting to phone you and visit you, but phoning is so impersonal and with the little ones, visiting also difficult for us. I want to reassure you that my thoughts and all my family's are with you and that we all wish from the bottom of our hearts for you to have a speedy painless recovery. I cannot express how sorry and sad I am that this should happen to you, but we believe that you will be fine. Please be strong and think positively because there is so much that can be done for you."

Michael's father sent postcards almost every day from his seaside home a thousand miles away.

"I hope you are feeling much better after your big chemo bash, relax and recover.
The chemo must be a trial for you, all very wearing. I am with you in it all of the ways that I can be. I wish you could get a few days down here. The weather has turned out very nice. Hold fast Michael. Life has long-term horizons as well as medium-type horizons. Never be horizonless."

And so many more . . .

"Sorry I missed you when I called. I am so very sorry about your illness. I do pray that God will be with you and give you many many days filled with blessings beyond belief. Our hearts are so encouraged by your progress . . . but more than that you have inspired us with your courage and your faithfulness."

"I pray that the Lord will touch your life with faith in Him with strength to endure. I pray that you have a full and fulfilling life in the years to come and will be blessed with a good wife."

"It is my prayer that you will feel his presence and seek comfort from Him who loves us so much. He is holding each one of us in the palm of His hand. 'What then shall we say in response to this? If God be for us, who can be against us.'"

The Purple Envelope

"It's very encouraging to see how positive you are. When you read scripture like Philippians chapter 4 verse 13, be sure of God's promises! Thinking of you while you're ill."

"Right now I'm sure life seems hard for you. But many prayers are being said for you and we know God hears our prayers. May He watch over you and keep you safe."

"We will keep you in our prayers. Hang in there, which is easier said than done. It makes me feel sad when you feel bad."

"Thinking of you in Christian love. We pray for you each and every day. We pray that you and your family draw strength from God almighty. May God give you a sense of peace Vivien. We thank God for your strength, love and commitment to Michael over the past year. We love you."

Composite love. How each one speaks to him in his own way. Not one more than another, just different facets of this thing called love. Tender, bold, exuberant, compassionate, patient expressions of love. A diamond has many facets, the sky has many stars, and no two are the same. Love is patient, love is kind. It isn't selfish and it always protects, always trusts and hopes, and it perseveres.

It is known that suffering produces perseverance which builds character. With character one has hope. And hope does not disappoint . . .

One lady wrote,

> "Your strength and courage make me ashamed of myself. Philippians chapter 4 verse 4. I love you lots."

Another expression of love in the form of a letter arrived one day in May. This one had an edge of urgency and almost a rebuke. Love has many facets and this man, his brother, cared deeply and brought this to him, and brought it in this way.

Michael read and pondered on what was written,

Hi Mike,

I am disappointed that you are making so little effort to be anointed with oil as in the scripture:

> "15 Is anyone among you sick? Let him call for the elders of the church, and let them pray over him, anointing him with oil in the name of the Lord. 16 And the prayer of faith will save the sick, and the Lord will raise him up." (James 5:15 & 16)

Also look at the following story (which you will know I'm sure):

> "10 And Elisha sent a messenger to him [Naaman the leper], saying, "Go and wash in the Jordan seven times, and your flesh shall be restored to you, and you shall be clean." 11 But Naaman became furious, and went away and said, "Indeed, I said to myself, 'He will surely come out to me, and stand and call on the name of the Lord his God, and wave his hand over the place, and heal the leprosy.'"

13 And his servants came near and spoke to him, and said, "My father, if the prophet had told you to do something great, would you not have done it? How much more then, when he says to you, 'Wash, and be clean'?" 14 So he went down and dipped seven times in the Jordan, according to the saying of the man of God; and his flesh was restored like the flesh of a little child, and he was clean." (2 Kings 5:10 – > 14) If I can compare this to your oncologist who prescribes months of side-effect inducing chemicals, which you accept and receive; yet the Bible tells you to do something which will take an evening max, and will leave you in need of a shower, and you shirk. Love you . . .

Michael considered all of this.

Many told him:

"Your courage is an inspiration to all of us.
  "Sorry you are having to go through this. We ask God to help you heal quickly."
  "Praying a song of praise to God will fill your soul with courage. There are no shortcuts to any place worth going."
  "You are in our thoughts and prayers. Your suffering is our own, your fears we share. Your hope is our hope. We love you and weep with you. God be with you, bestow you with His mercy and power while you see the example of your God and ours."

"Dear Michael,
We don't know each other very well but I've heard nothing but positive, loving comments made about you. You have a very wonderful family. You have been in my prayers and will continue to be so. I pray that God gives you the strength of mind to cope with your illness. May you continue to grow in faith daily. Your loving sister in Christ, Eve.

Another wrote:

'I haven't spoken much to you except for a greeting. However I have noticed you and seen a glow in you. You remind me of my son. I told him about you and he told me to tell you that he praises God that you are a child of God and if God allows, you might be going home soon. I cannot pretend to understand what you must be going through. I just want you to know that I care and that you would honour me if you ever wanted to talk to me. You are the age of my children. I know that only God can help us. God is in control.' In Christian Love . . .

These few greetings are a sample and there were many more – hundreds more.

"We are asking our Heavenly Father to be very close to you as you await the results of these long months of chemotherapy. You are so close to our hearts, we have grown spiritually because of the great faith you have shown – your courage. We love you.
                    Your church family."

I continue to watch these written gifts come in. All are different, and I see the giver more clearly than what he brings. Each one gives something that speaks to him in his own way – in a way of affection. Not one gift was more than any another – just different expressions of caring. Beside his bed is the potted Love Palm from a group of youngsters who were grinning as they came to his bed side.

"Flowers aren't cool for boys".

Their card said,

"No words that anyone can say will really ease the sadness and pain of your heart right now, but we hope it will comfort you in some small way to know that we care and are praying for you continuously."

12

"To put your life in danger from time to time breeds
a saneness in dealing with day to day trivialities.
Neville Shute

Michael was facing the prospect of high dose chemotherapy, but ordinary life went on. I was out of work and something that was important for us right then was that I could choose the hours in which I worked. I wrote to a magazine with an idea for an article that had been simmering for a while. They liked it and I went on to interview people in the lovely country area north west of Johannesburg. I photographed tea gardens and beautiful out of the way places for coffee stops and wrote up the articles. It was good to be talking to people about that which was their passion – easy and inspiring.

So it was that we came to this, the ultimate treatment. The term 'high dose' therapy was understood – a course of treatment that had a high level of toxins.
The outcome? The remaining stubborn cancer cells would be annihilated.

The side effects? His body would no longer be able to manufacture blood cells because of bone marrow damage. The bone marrow would then be regenerated by an infusion of healthy stem cells. They would migrate to the bone marrow spaces where they would grow.

Was it too desperate a measure? We were told there was a possible 50% chance of success. There was no alternative choice then, nothing else to try.

How awed we were by medical science. The process which was offered to Michael had been researched for years and the procedure finely tuned. Each patient to undergo it would no doubt add to the store of information for the future. Years ago they talked about doctors 'practising' medicine!

The success of this treatment depended very much on a supply of healthy stem cells, harvested either from a donor, or preferably from Michael himself. Even though Michael's body was depleted, youth is a positive factor and they would go ahead to get the required stem cells from him before considering the alternative of a donor.

Preparation for the process was made. There were more blood tests. They told us that among other things, they wanted to know that his heart was strong, that he was not HIV positive, and that he had not had glandular fever.

He was preparing to face the unknown yet again.

We both expected that there would be a day or two to get the stem cells from him, then four days for the high dose chemo. After that he'd get his stem cells back and it would all be over in a week or so.

How wrong we were.

There were delays and through them I noticed Michael in high spirits as if he felt a sense of freedom, as if on borrowed time, not having chemo after all. He had a considerable beard then, full eyebrows and eye lashes and lots of short blond hair on his head.

His stem cell count was taken to see how successfully they might get a sufficient harvest of cells from him before the high dose therapy. The blood test showed a low count and to raise it, a course of hormone injections was given. We did that at home.

All the time, fresh information came our way. We listened with surprise when told that the hormone we were using to boost his stem cell supply may have originated from the ovary of a Chinese rodent. Could that be right?

We wondered about many things in those days.

They did more chemo to up the stem cell production. This was an important part. By doing it in combination with a dose of chemo, the stem cells increased in rebound. With the help of this conditioning chemo the white blood cell count was kept low. He was soon given the go ahead for harvesting.

To make the harvesting process, as well as the administration of the high dose chemotherapy easy, a central catheter was inserted into a large vein near his heart. It was inserted with a local anaesthetic and the tubes came through a small hole in his skin near his collar bone. That foot long catheter would carry fluid, blood, the chemo-cocktail and medicines, and even make blood test samples easy to get to. There would be no more needles and searching for veins.

Michael was grinning as he told us that, from the beginning, he had counted the needles that were inserted into his veins, and he stopped counting, a while back, when it reached two hundred.

The tubes would stay in his chest until the full process of high dose chemotherapy and stem cell transplant were at an end.

Stem cell extraction began and the process was to be repeated at intervals of two weeks. Our regular Monday appointments were early at the unimposing building which was one of only two such centres in South Africa. It was fortunate that it was less than thirty minutes from home, and how good that Michael's medical insurance was financing it.

We walked in to the vital place with its high ceilings and high tech machinery. It seemed to us a cutting edge marvel of medical science and we were somewhat speechless at the explanation of what was happening.

The machine that separates the cells from the blood is a bit like those used in dairies to separate cream from milk using centrifugal force. It can separate platelets, plasma and, for these patients, it isolates the stem cells. Michael's blood was drawn into the machine. No more than a cup full of his blood was in the machine at one time, and was immediately returned to his body through the tube in his chest. The process of extraction took about four hours and so he settled down trustingly for the morning to submit to the process.

Between the visits, his production of stem cells continued to be stimulated by the hormone injections. The harvests were stored in small bags with a special preservative to prevent stem cell damage. Storage was at sub zero temperatures until needed. The objective was to extract sufficient stem cells and thankfully, after several Mondays, enough cells had accumulated from the extractions.

We remained aware of the importance of this preparation before high dose therapy. The marrow's function of blood cell production would start up again with these healthy stem cells when the highly toxic treatment was over. His own stem cells were the best replacement option and provided that they harvested sufficient of them, there would be no need for a donor. If he could not supply what was needed, the search for a compatible donor would begin with us – his family – before going to the national register of donors. The register was much like that of blood donors.

Another cancer patient was there. We met David, a boy with leukaemia. He waited, weak and unresponsive while his 15 year old brother Matt donated stem cells for him. The staff executed the administration quietly and with no fuss in the hall. Their professionalism was marked. Who can know the dynamics behind it?

The parents understood the process and the good fortune that their second son could, and was willing to, donate his stem cells. Matt's healthy bone marrow would naturally replace what he gave away. It is the normal process of life. The mother and father sat with their boys and gratefully saw light at the darkened end of a tunnel that was this cancer patient's life.

Michael's stem cells were transported to reach the lab department of the South African National Blood Service (SANBS). It was in our locality, and was the only stem cell bank in South Africa then. At the lab the stem cells were stored at -197^0C and could remain in storage for years before being used for a transplant. His would remain there until the request came from his doctor that he was ready for the infusion.

The people in those labs are effectively the back room guys in this wonderful life saving process. For speed and cleanliness, they work closely with the doctor. They personally collect and deliver the stem cells. Nothing is left for a delivery service so there's no delay in the process either between the harvest and the SANBS, or from there to the hospital.

Finally they were satisfied with the supply of his stem cells. It was time to go ahead with the high dose treatment.

Michael received the high doses of chemo by means of the catheter in his chest. He was admitted to a ward for this process so that his condition, especially his liquid intake, could be monitored to protect his kidneys from damage.

In my home in the evenings of that week I wrote often, especially to Belinda. Far away in Tampa she showed interest in the details and handled my need to communicate at these times.

Dear Belinda,

Thank you for emailing on a day that was so full for you. It has been a week of bravery for Michael. I say that because he has submitted himself to treatment that is highly stressful for his body. The nurses pay great attention to his liquid intake (and passing) and take trays of tea to him constantly because he will drink that more readily than the water. Their concern is that the kidneys continue to function well with the chemotherapy. Last night I saw him looking rather flushed and obviously full of liquid. This morning – back to normal. Today should be the last of the chemo. Then two days rest . . .

Belinda was wonderfully supportive, and it all went on with emails. Her work was with a church in Florida and bulletins were circulated in which there were updates and requests for prayer.

In the two days rest period at home, he went in daily for blood tests until the white blood cell count dropped showing that he had no immune system. It was then time to return to hospital for his own stem cells to be put back in. The timing of this process was critical.

Doctor Mac called the lab in advance for delivery of the stem cells. They were still frozen in the small bags and were thawed in a warm water bath. A delivery time was given and the lab staff could assume that Michael would get his pre-med (which included antihistamine) thirty minutes earlier. At the doctor's call, the lab staff knew they must get the stem cells to him on time or his patient would die. They made a timely delivery and the infusion took place through the catheter.

It is an extreme procedure from the time that stem cells are harvested and the body receives the powerful treatment of high dose therapy, to the state of none immunity and recharge with stem cells in the bone marrow transplant ward. This treatment process is quite something to go through. Yes it is quite something for those people who have been 'there and back'.

13

There is an appointed time for everything,
And there is a time for everything under heaven.
Ecclesiastes 3v1

With his own stem cells infused back in him, Michael stayed in isolation to wait for stem cells to grow first and then white blood cells. We knew that he had cold baths with "Savlon" and that he had a soft bacteria free diet, but visiting was limited and so we saw none of it and didn't know a lot about what it was like for him there.

He simply said, "I was sick until my white blood cell was right and I felt normal again. Drinking anything was terrible and for seven days I had a constant fever. I had visits from Mom, Anthony – and Brenda visited once. I came back to have the tubes removed afterwards. Having them inserted into the vein near my heart, relieved me of all the injections."

We who visited him came one at a time, first scrubbing up with a hand and face wash and removing outer garments before getting clothed in sterile gowns, plastic over-shoes, and hair caps. We wore face masks, and brought no gifts. No plants or flowers were allowed.

The isolation ward was brand new – a very recently completed addition to the hospital.

Greatly to be appreciated was Henri the nurse, and we soon heard about his hobby – building model planes. If his approach to his work was stoic, his enthusiasm for modelling wasn't. He was flat-footed and heavy rather than overweight so his heaviness rather veiled his personality than his intellect. He was a great companion for Michael while nursing him through days of fever, when drinking was difficult, but essential. And when we visited, he was a great informant for us.

With the emphasis on keeping a germ free environment it was surprising to see Michael's own grubby shoes lying untouched under his bed from the day he was admitted. There was a reason for everything and so I didn't question it. We were just glad of the wonder hand and face wash that made it safe for Michael to have visitors in his room at all.

A chart on the wall outside his ward indicated his cell production. We checked it day after day and saw only a hand drawn line at zero level getting longer each day. Eight days, nine days, ten . . . and then we were ecstatic to see a slight rise above zero.

"Don't tell him yet," it was Henri speaking.

"Wait . . . just to be sure."

We held our breath and the following day it was showing a more significant rise. That's when Michael was told the good news – and was told he could go home.

It was over.

Over.

It was hard to grasp.

We had waited so long, and now it's over?

I searched Henri's face for reinforcement.

He nodded.

Yes, it's quite something to go through . . . for the people who have been 'there and back'.

For Michael, it is all over.

We packed his few things and took the lift down. We passed reception and the café for the last time. It was where I had so often walked to stretch my legs – where I might drink coffee or fresh orange juice and see people come and go – a cross-section of the community who wander in and out. They were local people such as you might see in a shopping mall or airport, but here they carried a different load – whether the visit spoke life or death, they were intent on their particular destination somewhere inside the hospital . . . and we were walking out of those swing doors, walking as if on air to the car park for the last time.

Everyone's life is a story and all this happened in one year of Michael's life. His story is unique just as everyone else's is. However, others will have walked similar paths. Many courageous people walk the streets and we do not know we walk alongside heroes – people with unseen scars.

There will always be appreciation for the work of medical scientists, for the part that their work plays in giving a chance for life, to so many.

At times like these Emily sent light-hearted emails for him. 8th July she wrote,

Hey Mig, How are you doing? Is it nice to be home from horspital? Mom said they took the pipe out of your chest. Severe. No more chick-sympathy to be gleaned from that little accessory, unfortunately. Mom also said your stem cell count is picking up. That's really good. I am so glad.

What is the drill now for you? Do you still stay away from people and bath in Dettol etc? How long for? I am so glad – I really have a good feeling that things are just going to get better for you now. Write back and tell me some stories, rory.

From: Michael 8 July

It is nice to be home, but I'm not feeling that great. I don't have the pipe, but I have the hole in the chest. I think this is better, as it looks less gross than a pipe.

My counts are in the normal range again, but I am to be careful for a few days. I also have a stomach bug which I need to toss. Had at one point, three different strong anti-biotics in one day, so I need to sort that out. Once my chest has healed as well, then I can go back to sleeping and driving normally. I think that after this weekend, things will be more normal again.

The male nurse in isolation is a bigger airplane buddy than me. He was telling me of the plastic model kits he put together. I cut out the pieces and stuck them together on mine. He cuts pieces out of his then sticks back on so the cockpit opens etc. Also takes a file and knife and gives his aircraft realistic flak damage. If the damage falls over an engine he paints the engine black etc.

From: Emily July 9

Hey. Sorry you're not feeling great. I think you will soon. Maybe not soon like in five minutes, but I think it will be all upwards for you now. Where is the hole in your chest? Will it leave a scar or a hole like a bullet hole? Chicks dig scars.

I am just glad you are starting to recover. I know you are going to be fine, and I still have the picture of being at your wedding in a couple of years.

Interesting about the male nurse.

Hey, it could have been a small bullet hole where the pipe was. A girl would not know the difference.

Arrghh. It is a bit sad – I weigh about 68kg and am shorter and smaller boned than you and you are 67kg. I am obviously more chunky than you – have decided to take this in hand. You will put all that muscle back on in time. Hopefully I will lose all this lard in no time.

How are you doing today? How are you feeling?

Today I went to this place where you pick your own strawberries and raspberries. I only bothered with raspberries as there were more of them and they were easy to pick. It was such a brilliant day – all farm sounds and warm sun. I ate a few as well but burnt some calories too. It is odd that you have to be soooo thin to be the same weight as me NOT soooo thin. I would like to be thinner than I am, but I don't think about it a lot.

Tell me some things.

Michael replied July 10,
Hmmm, odd that I have to be SOOO thin, with match-stick legs etc to weigh the same as you.

14

> I fly because it releases my mind
> from the tyranny of petty things.
> Antoine de Saint-Exupery

With Michael back home after the successful bone marrow functioning, I was cautiously elated. We planned a trip to the coast, a holiday to shake off the malaise of months of tending to low level existence that had hope but no proven assurance for the future.

Michael was gaining weight and hair growth. He had life. Then why was it hard to get closure. My dogged spirits seemed to have settled in.

There was no halting his progress . . .

But, it was not over.

It was put to him that where the cancer had started, there remained a shrunken lump of dead cancerous cells. It may dissipate over time, but if one live cell existed, its re-growth could not again be fought with chemo. Would he choose to have the remnant surgically removed, or left for the body to naturally clear away.

Many onlookers offered their opinions. Leave well alone, was a popular one. I had had enough . . . as had Michael.

I wrote to Emily, August 05, 2002:

> We had a good chat with the surgeon who said that it is surgically possible to remove the lesion but it is not in the easiest of places. He showed it to us on the scan (I've not seen it before). It is actually about two and one half inches in diameter and is nestled in between his backbone, aorta, renal vein, and near the stomach and a kidney. What the surgeon cannot know before he opens up is whether it is firmly stuck to any of the above things or just lightly attached. He said that after so much aggressive chemotherapy, this remnant will be encased in hard concrete-like stuff. There may be a bunch of malignant cells nestling in it, or not. He told us that it's an oncological decision not a surgical one and outlined what to expect from the operation if it's what Michael chooses.

Around this time I was feeling some strain. Michael was approving the recovery path and his choices were sometimes hard to navigate. I was facing the possibility of the operation with great reluctance and was hardly a support to him. It was sorted out though, this time partly with the help of a note that I left on the counter for him as I went out early to an interview.

> Michael, I am really sorry for what I said last night. I am sorry because it probably wasn't helpful

although it was intended to be. Remember I am on your side, and here for you, while you get the framework of your life in order again. I may sometimes need help to know what your need is, but I always love you. Can we work towards me having the few days in Ballito? Come too, or I will arrange whatever's needed for you for that week, if you would rather stay behind.

* * *

Our trip to the coast goes ahead along with Anthony and Tanya, and their girls. Ballito is relaxing – walks along the sand, finding sea shells, bathing in rock pools and spotting dolphins leaping through glimmering metallic blue sea. The girls judder along the board walk on their tricycles. For them it's an adventure and sand castles are built and broken down by the dozen. Moats around the sand castles are filled with sea water, and empty out with timeless inevitability.

While Anthony and Tanya have time to themselves, I settle down to read to their girls. Often they say,
"No Gran, tell us about the old days."
And so we begin with tales that they've heard before, of my mother's childhood – these South African girls who don't know snow, love to hear how their great grandmother raced down snow-covered slopes on trays smuggled from the kitchen – and got caught. They laugh about her bicycle ride down narrow Devonshire lanes that wind steeply, on a day when she met cows ambling along and her brakes failed. Then skipping-rope games that are often unfamiliar to a generation of children playing on computer keyboards.

The children sit closer; Carla climbs on my lap.

The Purple Envelope

And so I recall again some competitive fun I had with three brothers and a sister as well as the abandon of acrobatics and that practised poise of ballet, wearing sequined wings. I wonder how it is that these stories hold my grandchildren's attention no matter how often they hear them, and it seems that in telling them, some of the vitality I've lost of late is restored.

I pause and Carla slips off my lap and dances and from somewhere we hear Anthony calling.

Then comes the familiar sound of an approaching light aircraft and from the balcony we see it over the sea. Its flight follows the curve of the foam below. The girls wave excitedly as Michael flies past and he waves back. There's something normal about the afternoon, marvellous normality.

We stay and watch birds hover like eagles that swoop to nab their prey. How like the North American Inuit who waits at a breathing hole. In flight these birds glide effortlessly until the moment to dive and seize a fish for lunch. The microlight flies a little higher than the birds. At five hundred feet one gets a bird's eye view not seen from larger planes.

Michael's plane has gone and we stay on the balcony and watch the sea and see nothing of the activity below its slightly ruffled surface. The Indian Ocean here is turquoise today but in the darkness of the deeper sea that's near the horizon, there's purple. Darkness does not always have a colour.

Here in its season comes the sardine run. Here too, sharks and dolphins. The sea does not of itself show what is concealed below, but man's curiosity takes him there and what he finds may fill him with wonder; may fill him with terror.

Below us is the boardwalk defining the line of land alongside sand dunes capped with succulents with showy purple flowers and sap that heals. Their green shoots grow like fingers holding the mounds of sand. Roots hold the sand so it doesn't slither onto the beach where it would be vulnerable to the relentless tidal rising and falling away of the sea as it yields to the pull of the moon. Wet sand has walkers' footprints on it, imprinting patterns until the next wave wipes away the indentations, leaving a tidy smooth floor.

A freak tornado hits the shore that night and does damage that's disruptive but repairable, and life goes on. Just as an upturned stone exposes mini life and flurried activity goes on until order is restored.

And in this neighbourhood I overhear artists and writers talk. They will paint and write here because this place inspires them. And Michael was inspired as his flight followed the curve of the foam below.

That is where he was when he decided to have the cancer's remnant surgically removed.

15

> "Child of God, you were born to manifest the glory of God which will liberate others to do so also"
> M Williamson

I rise from bed lightly but robotic because no decisions are mine to make. It's operation day. The minutes and hours for most people pass as normally as every other day. For us such a day has never been before.

We arrive at the hospital and the procedure is the same. The medical information exchange is steady, professional, efficient and kindly from the receptionist, nurse, sisters, and from the surgeon.

His mood speaks confidence cheerily. We're reassured as much by his manner as by his words. Everything is in place for a successful morning's work. I stare at him. He will make an eight inch cut down Michael's front from the base of his ribs. Through the opening he'll remove the lump of dead cancerous cells that are in his back, attached to his spine, aorta, renal vein and stomach. It's the place, just below his heart, where the tumor started.

I find a seat to wait. The corner bench seat isn't comfortable; the red fabric not attractive. I find a paper to read and wonder how the meaning of words I know, float around my comprehension. Nothing settles as my eyes pass over the words and I'm aware that none of the information will be available in my memory to be drawn on tomorrow or any other day.
"Hi there!"
Anna's warm melodious voice makes me look up and one, who is an acquaintance rather than friend, sits beside me.
"I thought you could use some company."
I smile appreciating her thoughtfulness while moving along the not too comfortable seat. Her cheerful easy chatter continues and time passes unnoticed. Yes her company is what I need. I appreciate her awareness and its spontaneous response. Her mood lightens the seriousness surrounding this morning and what it means to us.

Long after the time we expected the operation to be finished there is no sign of Michael. I sit alone after Anna leaves . . . and then I see him. Is it him?
A nurse is pushing the stretcher and he is grey.
He is so grey. Quickly on my feet I walk with them. I wonder about his grey pallor.
In the ward, the Sister states,
"It's an empty ward. There's a bed in here for you if – if you want to stay with him?"
"Stay? Oh yes."

The Purple Envelope

His seemingly lifeless body is shifted skilfully onto a bed. He sleeps. I see the dark head of the smiling handsome surgeon above the nurses as he arrives. The smile affirms his confidence as he states that all the cells are removed. Unquestioningly I trust. I will sleep here tonight.

The day passes. I see him in the bed next to mine and he knows I am here. He comes through the usual recovery from anaesthetic, and I wait. This shadow of a man is my son and all I can do is to wait. When you know that all you can do is be near; that's what you do – just stay nearby knowing comfort is what your presence evokes.

Now and again as he sleeps, I stretch my legs.

Long corridors are lined here and there with parked stretchers and trolleys. I don't take the lift, leave them for hospital use, and instead walk down a wide staircase, hand sliding along the hand rail finding the texture of wood pleasant in this place of sterile stainless steel and plastic. At a corner table in the coffee shop, I order coffee. Its aroma is enough but I drink it too.

Through the clear plastic overlay on the table, I read and read again a note next to my cup and saucer.

"Weeping may endure for a night, but joy comes in the morning."

I stir dark sugar into my coffee. It has been a long long night.

Today is 29th August.

It's a year since I had the call from Emily saying that Michael had cancer – the tumour was eight inches by six inches when it was discovered.

The next day brings visitors. Tanya comes. She sits in her usual place at the end of the bed. The intravenous morphine drip is administered by a button under Michael's left thumb. Tanya watches his thumb pulse on the button. The pain is considerable, especially when laughing. And yes he is really laughing.

After the disturbance that surgery causes, he hasn't eaten or drunk – not since the night before the operation. There is progress every day. A few sips of water on the first day, a cup of tea on day two, when he was also able to stand up with help. And on the third day he stood without help. We are waiting for the results of the lab tests on the lesion which will be through tomorrow.

He stays there for three days before going to a private ward. His visitors are the ones he has seen through all the stages of his physical struggle. The caring attention from church members was like family care for we who have no extended family in this country. Friends were daily around his bed. Their loyalty never flagged in any way.

Patio chairs, tables and sun umbrellas furnish the balcony leading from the private ward. I sip fresh orange juice through a straw while seated there, and my tapestry grows close to completion. Michael comes through the doors to join me; how good he looks. Nurses who saw him come out of the three hour operation come by and don't recognise him. He looks calm and relaxed and his face is composed with the blue eyes so clear behind clear skin and dark stubble. Amazing how his pallor and energy improves.

The sun shines overhead.
Michael will soon be home.
He is well.

I write to Emily who is still in England but who would have been beside her brother through it all if she could have been:

> I wish you could see him now, now it's over. He looks good and his friends have been great this week. Joe's Mom sells Justin skin products and she sent natural tissue oil for his scars. He has slept a lot and has eaten well. He's doing fine.

Emily's reply:

> Good about Michael's friends. Who could believe this would go on for over a year. It is one year since I flew over with the boys, and now Leon starts school.

Tests show that there was no life in the remnant – except for a small area next to the aorta that had the potential to grow again. Specialist physician medical oncologists say he had a retroperitoneal germ cell tumor, with lung metastases, treated with combination chemotherapy including peripheral blood stem rescue, with surgical removal of inactive non-malignant tumour tissue thereafter.

Michael leaves hospital and leaves behind all traces of cancer. Thirty four staples from his chest to his stomach will be removed to leave slight scarring.

We are nearing the end. Michael is over the last stage of his treatment! Rarely have so few words held such meaning for me. The reality of recovery penetrates my mind but my heart must wake from its emotional slumber. He stands there with eyebrows and hair now returning. Not the greatest picture of health, but a man with resolve.

He leaves the hospital for the last time, but he'll be back to the outpatients for three monthly routine tests. It is over and it shows in the way he walks. It shows in that silent resolve that is so typical of Michael.

* * *

It's a long time since he started this journey of recovery. The time came for me to write a letter to the many people who made up the backdrop of our lives.

10.10.02
Dearest Friends,

I started to write this letter quite a few times during the past several months. Each time I was seeing Michael take a step towards recovery. Always there followed a new course of treatment and each seemed more harsh than the last. And now, with a year of treatment behind him, I can write this letter fully to tell you of our gratitude for each thought and prayer, each note and text message, every smile and every hug.

Thank you, from Michael and all his family, for the love you showed us that was always both kind and cheerful. We felt your gentle compassion and were encouraged to persevere with hope and trust.

We are thankful that in this way, we could feel your hand in ours along the way,

And we are thankful for the skill of the medical team.

The Purple Envelope

I sometimes look across at Michael and am reminded that God is gracious to us and we can attribute the glory and honour to Him.

God bless you.

Our love always.
Vivien and Michael

. . . there is indeed nothing new under the sun; whenever I read Philippians chapter 2 verse 27 I will be reminded of these days.

16

> Whoever you are: step out of doors tonight,
> out of the room that lets you feel secure.
> Infinity is open to your sight.
> R.M. Rilke

Independence was important to Michael. For so long he had been dependent on the process, the doctors and others. He said it was important that he search himself and his own life – as if needing to reclaim it. After so many doctors and people telling him what to do to survive, there was a need to decide for himself about his life – what to do.

He wrote to his cousin:

Hi Sarah,
    It has been a very long time since I have written. I am sorry about that. Not too much has happened though. Most of my life was involved in spending a few days at work, then spending a few days getting chemo – or so it seemed. I know my mom told you

about us going to Ballito. I managed to get some flying done while there, first time in ages.

It seems like my battle with C is coming to a close. I shall be making an appointment with my oncologist shortly, as enough time since the operation has passed. My stomach has healed quite well, and I am able to move about fairly easily. I'm not very flexible though. Had a small incident where I had to go back to hospital for a few days after the op, but it was nothing serious.

We shall see what steps need to be taken next. I am quite frustrated though as it has been drawn out so far. Remember we were first hoping that it would be over by Dec/Jan? Back then I thought I might come to the UK in June but I have been unable to get a look at coming over because of the uncertainty involved with the treatment. As soon as I had recovered a bit from a course of chemo, I had to go back to it.

Thankfully I had a break before the op, while I was deciding whether to go ahead with it or not, but had to say 'NO!' to the op before I could relax again, which I did not. I am sorry I have been so quiet regarding this issue, but please understand that I have had too much uncertainty. I am hoping to come and visit later on this year, or more likely early half of next year – might even try to get a job there for a while . . . to annoy everyone ☺.

I hope I might get the odd photo of your travels. You must have had an amazing time, and be much the wiser for it. I am quite jealous of you being able to travel like that. I met an Israeli girl in Durban who has been travelling for a year, was up in Iceland

and since then has been travelling through Africa. What a life.

My hair has grown back, fallen out and grown back again. I shall hopefully have some pictures soon that I can send. Love Michael.

And so some normality returns.

Gaby calls, exuberantly happy with us for the results, and says that in her consultation with Michael before his treatment started, she asked him what he saw for himself in five years time.

"Viv, he immediately answered 'flying my microlight'. He saw his future, and I knew he was in the right frame of mind for survival. He would recover."

Yes he was over the last stage of his treatment; the very last stage and life began to return to normal.

We are waiting no more.

Waiting is replaced, quite suddenly, with activity. Can he take all this activity so soon?

In the new normality, he introduced new things. The first came two weeks later in the form of fencing. An old school friend invited him along.

After the debilitating process that he'd come through, could such a demanding sport possibly be appropriate! Perhaps there are few other activities so well suited to his condition. If like me you don't know the sport beyond viewing sword combats enacted in film scenes, usually for historic moments of valour, romance, or revenge, this is a highly physical and mental activity. Speed, strength, focus and perception of the opponent's intent, followed with a fast response, are some of the characteristics of the sport.

So it was that Michael joined a fencing club and faced those challenges. Each session ended with his shirt, worn inside a garment made of tough cloth that didn't allow for the body to breathe, being soaking wet. I happily pushed them into the washing machine – shirts that were wet with perspiration and I imagined that those fencing bouts helped to detoxify him and sharpen his thinking.

It was spring time in Johannesburg as he began his life in this way. Most important of all, he was having fun and that love for a challenge with a competitive edge was stimulated again.

About that time, Michael again remarked on the change in his taste buds. No longer enjoying sweet things, he stopped drinking cola, and found a taste for beer. The water he drank was from a jug that had fresh lemon slices in it.

The fencing lasted for months and then canoeing became the new interest, and the mastery of balance, rhythm, coordination and synergy. The outcome of failing to maintain this was a dip in cold water and a swim to the shore of the dam. That's when his t-shirts came to the washing machine, wet with dam water.

Cricket was Michael's favourite game, and it began again for him with a new local team – and was such easy fun. Supporters at their casual club matches, watched as some of the men pulled shirts out of their bags that varied from grey to mottled cream. Not all were ironed and some pants were crumpled and stained in varying degrees with grass.

Their ages were from fifteen to fifty, and Michael fitted in, happy in a way that made us smile just to see. It wasn't about playing top league class games. It was about having fun within the bounds of the rules. Their natural sense of competition ruled and improved their game so that with their wonderful team spirit, within a year they progressed up the league.

I have to imagine the fencing and rowing, the long distance running, cycling, swimming and indoor cricket, played a part in a fuller recovery. In those months of regeneration, there was also badminton, squash and a bungee jump at Bloukrans.

Bloukrans is near the Tsitsikamma Forest Village Market and the jump there is from the world's highest single span concrete bridge. While on the Cape Province's Garden Route, Michael drove past it and had a spontaneous thought,

"If I am going to bungee once in my life I may as well make it the highest in the world."

He wore a full body harness and the jump took him down 216 meters from the bridge to the surface of the river's water.

But a trip to see the sun's eclipse had advanced planning involved. Afterwards he told us, "We drove to the north of South Africa to catch the eclipse. There were six of us in the car and we drove into the area where it would happen. There we slept in a tent at the side of the road and caught it perfectly in the morning; the total eclipse of the sun. Wonderful."

These things were all part of his journey back to where he had been – the studying too was resumed. And before too long we decided to move house – we were, after all, having a new start.

I sensed that a lovely girl that came into our lives mattered very much on his road to full recovery.

The Purple Envelope

Three monthly blood checks confirmed that he remained free from cancer. As he heard positive results from those blood checks, his smile showed the relief he felt and he began to welcome the tests for the confirmation they gave. That full smile of his, we had not seen for a very long time.

Marie and Gill, the oncology nurses noticed a change in him too.

"I get goose bumps to see him walk back in here," one said.

"It's as if he's a different person. As a chemo patient, he was quiet, almost unnoticeable, as if blending into the background. Today I see a change in his personality – with that sense of humour – he's so funny! It is good to see him well and thriving."

He was back.

He had, against such odds, remarkably become a cancer survivor, and I am reminded of the written words I sent in a purple envelope from a small English Post Office.

I wish you a life in which you fly,
in which you soar in your endeavours.

And yes, a lovely girl came into his life so that, just as she had pictured it, Emily was at her brother's wedding. It was seven years after his recovery, and there are people who say they will remember it especially for its tenderness . . .

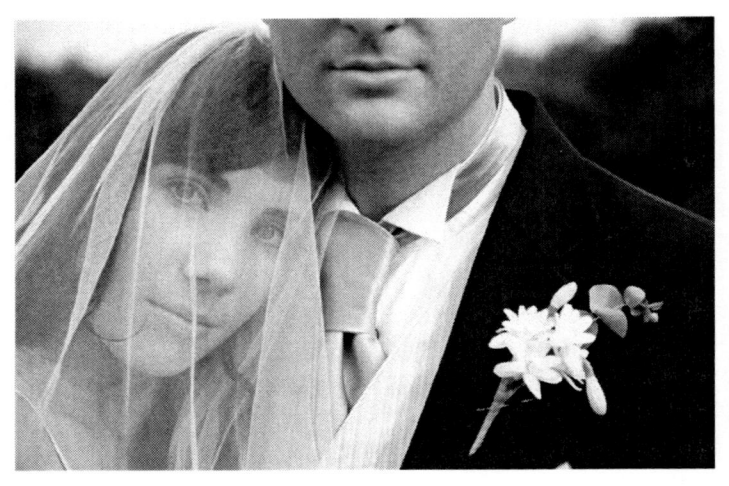

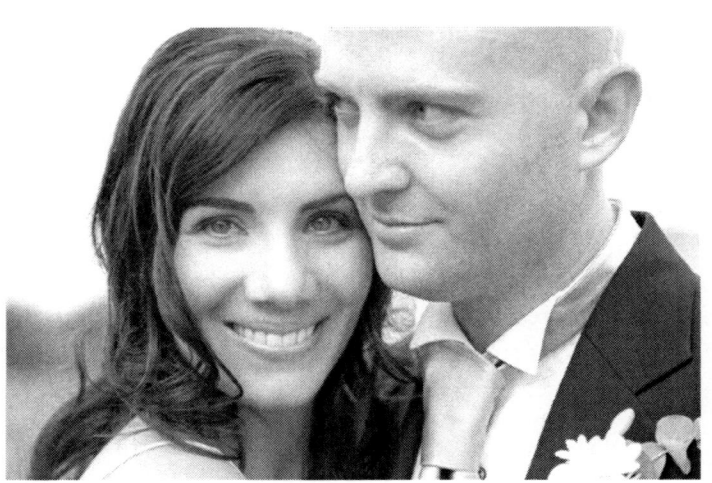

The Purple Envelope

From the Preachers pen:

"About two years ago, one young man in the congregation, by the name of Michael James, was diagnosed with inoperable cancer.

He was just twenty years old.

I had known Michael for fifteen years – ever since I began preaching in that congregation. One day, after Michael told me about his condition – he confided in me that the specialist told him that there was no hope and he would not live to see Christmas – this was in August. He said his stomach was rock hard with the growth, and he could not keep down any food.

He asked me to put my hand on his stomach and as I did so, I could feel the enormous growth which had invaded his body.

Not only was Michael devastated by his impending death, but the whole church agonized with him.

One thing that constantly amazed me though about Michael, was his strength of faith. Never once did I ever hear him complain that he had a raw deal. Did he complain or grumble to anyone that at 20 years old he was going to miss out on so much life?

He went to another specialist who said to him that though his condition was not operable, he could try some method of treating the cancer. The cancer is a type that afflicts mainly young men up to 30 years of age. Michael underwent a radical chemotherapy treatment that would have overwhelmed many men. But still Michael's faith was without falter.

The elders were asked if we would anoint him with oil in accordance with James chapter 5 verses 14, 15. Some might eschew the idea as outdated and mystical – but . . .

On a quiet weekday morning, the elders gathered together at the church building and met with Michael. In a moving prayer chain – each offered up to God a prayer on Michael's behalf – entreating the Father to have mercy upon Michael. Then each one at a time poured a little oil on his hands and laid his hand on Michael's head.

Michael's faith in God and in the Scripture, together with a whole new eating plan and intensive chemotherapy and I believe with strengthening from prayer, did something in Michael's life.

Initially Michael was given less than three months to live. The cancer had spread throughout his lungs and through the course of his treatment, he became nothing more than skin and bone, and disease.

A year later, Michael was pronounced free of all the cancer, and he remains a strong and faithful Christian and a blessing to all who know him.

Bob Pearce

* * *

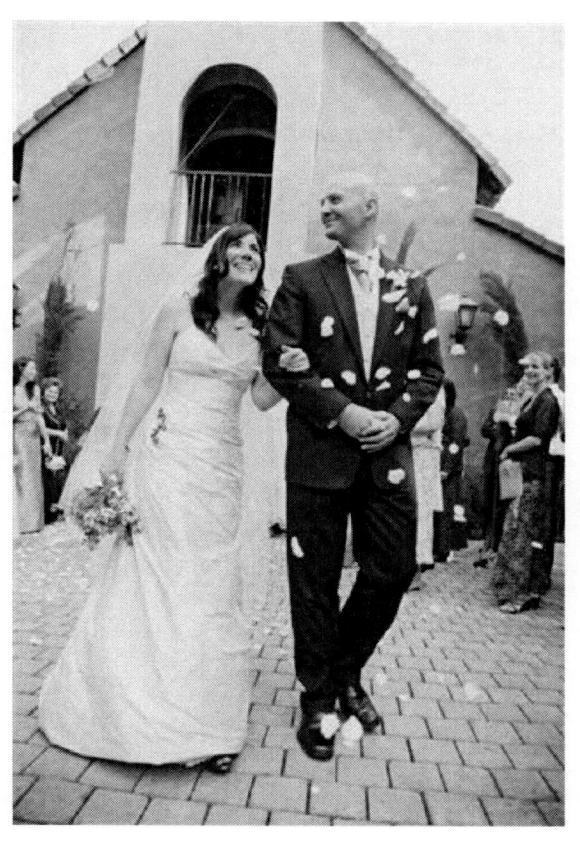

Life's Flight

Fly with me and take the sky
It is now that my life is mine.
I've got this short time on earth
And my longing has brought me here.
All I lacked and all I gained
And yet it's the way that I chose.
My trust was far beyond words.
That has shown me a little bit
Of the heaven I have found.
I want to feel that I'm alive
All my living days.
I want to feel that I'm alive,
Knowing it was good enough.
Anon

Bibliography

Chemotherapy and I by D. Lumley

Dead doctors don't lie.

Challenge Cancer the Holistic way.
By Monica Fairall

Eat right for your type [blood type]
By Dr Peter J.D'Adamo

I have Cancer - A Message of Hope
By Helfried HR Crede

Beating Cancer
By Dr Willem Serfontein

Spring Clean your System
By Jane Garton

Whole energy - health foods one by one
By Caryl Vaughan-Scott

Your Body's Many Cries for Water.
By Dr F. Batmangheligj

Vivien Jones

The Chemotherapy & Radiation Therapy Survival Guide
By Judith McKay, Nancee Hirano

A Himalayan Trinity. Part 1 - A House in Higher Hills
By Mark Kingsley

The Bible

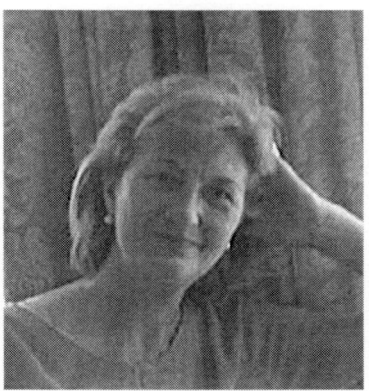

Vivien Jones

Vivien was born in Bristol, England and from teaching in East Anglia she moved, with her husband, to South Africa. Her experiences there were with cerebral palsied adults and in counseling. Many of those years were spent as a housewife, but later on, marketing, photography and conservation supported her life both in South Africa and England.

Vivien's varied life equips her to tell of a range of responses that are evoked when the cards that are dealt are tough. Cancer was new to her when it came uninvited into her family. To add to what the professionals were doing, she delved into other aspects of recovery, learning of medical procedures and nutritional needs and much more that would support healing and stimulate full recovery.

Vivien has three children and four grandchildren and if you ask her about herself, that's what she will begin by telling you.

Lightning Source UK Ltd.
Milton Keynes UK
UKOW050555041111

181444UK00001B/31/P